Where Have My Eyebrows Gone?

One Woman's Personal Experiences with Chemotherapy

Best wishes —

Maureen

Mc Cutcheon

Where Have My Eyebrows Gone?

One Woman's Personal Experiences with Chemotherapy

Maureen McCutcheon, R.N., B.S.N., M.Ed.

Illustrations by Kelly McCutcheon, B.A.

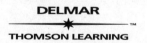

DELMAR

TM

THOMSON LEARNING

Australia Canada Mexico Singapore Spain United Kingdom United States

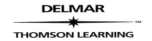

DELMAR

THOMSON LEARNING ™

Where Have My Eyebrows Gone? One Woman's Personal Experiences with Chemotherapy
by Maureen McCutcheon

Business Unit Director:
William Brottmiller

Executive Marketing Manager:
Dawn F. Gerrain

Art/Design Coorindator:
Robert Plante

Project Development Manager:
Marion S. Waldman

Editorial Assistant:
Robin Irons

Project Editor:
David Buddle

Project Development Editor:
Jill Rembetski

Illustrator:
Kelly McCutcheon

Project Coordinator:
Nina Lontrato

Library of Congress
Cataloging-in-Publication Data

McCutcheon, Maureen.
    Where have my eyebrows gone? :
one woman's personal experiences
with chemotherapy / Maureen
McCutcheon ; illustrations by
Kelly McCutcheon.
    p. cm.
    ISBN 0-7668-3934-6
    1. Breast--Cancer--Chemotherapy--
Popular works.   I. Title.
    RC280.B8 M3564 2001
    616.99'449061--dc21
                          2001042521

NOTICE TO THE READER

Dedication

This book was written as a tribute to those women who have chosen to fight the good fight against one of the most feared diseases that women face—breast cancer—and to the surgeons, oncologists and oncology nurses who help them do that.

My wig is off to each and every one of them.

CONTENTS

Preface

I wrote *Where Have My Eyebrows Gone?* for women who are coping with chemotherapy after surgery for breast cancer. I hope this book will inform and encourage these women by helping them understand the nature of cancer, chemotherapy and the symptoms that may accompany treatment. Through this book, the reader will be encouraged to call upon her sense of humor, identify with me and deal with her symptoms during and immediately following the course of therapy with a more optimistic and enlightened view. The information about chemotherapy and resulting symptoms contained in this book can be applied to all women being treated with the same anticancer drugs as I took, not just those with breast cancer.

I am a registered nurse who has undergone chemotherapy following a lumpectomy then a mastectomy for breast cancer. The medical information in the book is based on my professional experience and research. Although not a textbook, it includes data from an oncology physician and an oncology nurse practitioner. The central theme of the book is my knowledge, views and experiences. Some of the latter are outrageous, some ludicrous. But be forewarned. Any or all of them could happen to you.

Information about symptoms and suggestions on how to deal with them are presented in a lighthearted way. Chemotherapy kills cancer cells but not sense of humor. Laughter and a positive attitude ease stress and lighten the spirit for the patient and her family and friends. Incorporating a sense of humor into chemotherapy makes the experience easier and more manageable for all. Laughter lengthens life and certainly makes it more enjoyable.

Many terms used to describe the symptoms experienced during chemotherapy graphically describe body functions. I have chosen to use nonclinical names that may appeal more to readers and that will inject humor into a situation that is anything but funny.

Short verses have been interspersed throughout the text for the enjoyment of the reader and to shift the focus to a lighter vein. For example

Cancer sucks but living is fun
Thank goodness chemo will soon be done.

My daughter, Kelly McCutcheon, an illustrator and graphic designer, has provided the cartoon-like drawings and a pattern for the book's design.

So, here's to life and laughter with the three big Cs: cancer, chemo and "cure!"

Acknowledgments

I wish to thank Dr. Joanna M. Brell, formerly of the Cleveland Clinic Health System, and currently with the Ireland Cancer Center of the Case Western Reserve University. She is my medical oncologist and hematologist. Her professional and compassionate care and her positive attitude inspire calm and courage to those to whom she ministers. She's a winner!

Also, my thanks go to Dr. Lawrence Levy and Dr. Randall Yetman, both of the Cleveland Clinic Health System. They are at the top of my list as breast surgeon, and reconstruction surgeon respectively.

Another member of my medical team to whom I am grateful is Dr. Terence Kilroy. He is an educator, a brilliant medical practitioner and a pulmonologist extraordinaire. Thanks, Doc, for helping me to remain on this earth.

Special thanks to Marion Waldman, Project Development Manager at Delmar Thomson Learning, for recognizing the value of this project and for her unyielding encouragement. And to Jill Rembetski, Project Development Editor, who contributed immeasurably to the evolution of this manuscript. She is a special talent and it was my pleasure to work with her.

I am especially grateful to Joanna Brell, MD and Barbara Tripp, RN for their knowledgeable contributions to this manuscript. This book is better for their participation.

Another special thank you goes to Lisa Silipo. She is a member of the Delmar team who contributed her own story about her experiences with breast cancer. She is a brave and courageous young woman who volunteered to contribute her insights to a project that she feels is of value.

Thanks also to the professional staff who helped turn this manuscript into a book. I appreciate their able assistance in the development, preparation and publication of this project.

I would also like to thank the following individuals for reviewing various drafts of the manuscript and for offering me suggestions for improvement: Jennifer French, Averill Park, NY; Mara Ginsberg, President, To Life, Breast Cancer Education & Support, Delmar,

NY; Ann-Marie Loscalzo, Leeds, NY; Barbara Sherman, Round Lake, NY; Peggy Smith, Sarasota, FL; Lisa Silipo, Albany, NY; and Melissa A. Longo, Brewster, NY.

I especially want to thank my daughter, Kelly McCutcheon, for the time and effort she expended to create the illustrations and consult on the graphic design and for sharing her creative ideas about content. Her drawings look amazingly like me—both with and without hair.

In addition, I thank those special people in my life who offered continuing encouragement and emotional support throughout my bouts with cancer as well as my adventures with chemotherapy and wig wearing. Special family members include Ruthanne and Jim Dillhoefer, Peg and Jack McCarthy, Maureen and Kevin McCarthy and Maureen Schubert. Special friends include Connie Kolleda, Barbara Gustafson, Mercita Fitzgerald, Joan Riess, Carol Litzler, Barbara Stepanek, Barbara Soltis, Joan Cikra and Tricia Marquard.

Individual accolades go to Maureen Lewis, my 38-year-old niece, who shared her surgical, chemo and life experiences with me. She juggled her job, husband, small children, home, surgery and chemo successfully. She's more than a trooper. She's my hero.

And, finally, I am thankful to and for my greatest treasures, my children—Kelly, my illustrator and graphic designer; Casey, my son, attorney and chief advisor; Kate, my world traveler and anthropologist; and Michael Simons, Kelly's husband, archeologist and my favorite (and only) son-in-law at this writing. They are my staunchest advocates and most significant legacy.

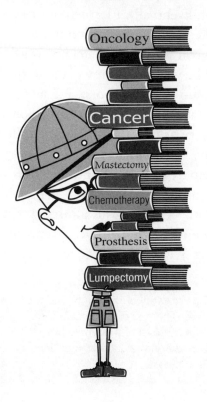

What's Up with Cancer and Chemotherapy?

I found my own breast cancer while doing a breast self-exam. There it was, directly under my right nipple. Of course, I denied that it was an actual tumor because I had been given a clean bill of health after my mammogram three months before. Also, there was no history of breast cancer in my family. So what was up with that lump, I wondered.

I searched repeatedly for a matching lump on the left side, hoping to confirm my "enlarged gland" theory. But no match could be found.

I had experienced occasional shooting pains in the right breast that confirmed my opinion that this lump could not be malignant. That's because I thought that cancer was not painful in its early stages. And the lump itself was not painful. So I felt comfortable waiting to see if that lump would go away under its own steam. It didn't. It got larger. Eventually, I learned not to wait for pain to have a lump checked but to have all lumps checked. I took myself off to a breast surgeon who immediately biopsied the lump there in his office. He said he would send my tissue to the lab to confirm the diagnosis, but suspected the worst. He suspected cancer and recommended that surgery be performed as soon as possible. I scheduled it that very day for the first moment he had free.

The surgeon gave me a choice, lumpectomy or mastectomy. His choice was mastectomy to be sure all cancer cells were removed. But because no lumps were palpable in the lymph glands under my arm, I chose the lumpectomy. I was informed that the statistics on recurrence were about the same between removing only the lump or the whole breast. We agreed on the lumpectomy.

> **LUMPECTOMY:** The removal of the tumor and the edges of the surrounding normal tissue. The rest of the breast is left in place.
> **MASTECTOMY:** The removal of the whole breast. This may involve removing the lymph nodes in the underarm to determine if the cancer cells have spread out of the breast.

Cancer Overview

The surgeon explained that cancer is a malignant tumor that has the ability to spread. The word *cancer* means "wild growth of cells." In other words, for some unknown reason, a few cells in one organ of the body all of a sudden begin to grow more rapidly than the adjacent cells. These cancerous cells invade the space that belongs to the normal cells of that organ. In fact, they devour the normal cells and take their place.

> **CANCER:** An uncontrolled growth of new and abnormal cells that invade surrounding tissue and can spread to other sites in the body. If left untreated, it is life threatening.
> **BENIGN TUMOR:** A new growth of abnormal tissue that remains in one site. It is not life threatening. It is not cancer.
> **MALIGNANT TUMOR:** A new growth of abnormal tissue that can spread throughout the body. It is life threatening. Cancer is an example of a malignant tumor

To make matters worse, cancer cells do not carry out the function of the cells they replace. They are just parasites on that organ. The cancer pushes the normal cells out of the way and devours some. That explained my shooting pains in the breast tissue, although it must be remembered that not all women have those shooting pains to draw their attention to a lump.

I learned that a major concern with cancer is that those fast-growing cells have the capacity to spread to other parts of the body where they repeat their fast-growing and devouring ways. Cancer spreads through the circulatory system. In other words, one cell breaks off from the cancerous tumor that is growing out of control, slips into the circulation and travels to another organ that offers a friendly environment. There, the cancer cell pops out of the vessel that carried it there, attaches itself to that organ and begins to grow and replace normal cells. This cancer is said to have metastasized. Exactly which cells will begin this process and why they grow so fast and spread to other organs is unknown and unpredictable.

The fact that cancer cells grow much faster than do normal cells in the body is good news and bad news. The good news is that because of their rapid rate of growth, the cancer cells can be treated. The bad news is that unless the cancer is detected early, those cancer cells can metastasize; that is, they can grow in a number of places in the body, invade normal cells and take over those organs. Early detection is the key to successful treatment.

Diagnostic Tests

PHYSICAL EXAM: A manual palpation of breast tissue to determine tumors, thickened areas and other physical changes.

MAMMOGRAM: An x-ray of breast tissue to detect abnormal growths before they can be felt.

COMPUTERIZED AXIAL TOMOGRAPHY (CAT) SCAN: A noninvasive test that uses x-ray and a computer to visualize transverse layers of body tissue.

MAGNETIC RESONANCE IMAGING (MRI): A noninvasive test that visualizes internal organs using powerful magnetic fields.

ULTRASOUND OR **SONOGRAM** is a test that uses inaudible sound waves to outline the shape of body organs.

As cancer cells grow they form lumps or tumors. Often these tumors can be felt or seen on x-rays, CAT scans, MRIs and ultrasound or sonography images. Some blood tests can indicate that cancer might be affecting certain organs such as the prostate gland. Unfortunately at this writing, there is no specific blood test for breast cancer.

If left untreated, cancer cells continue to replicate, travel to other organs and render them incapable of functioning. This process saps the energy of the person affected. If the cancer spreads to vital organs and renders them nonfunctional, the person dies. That is why cancer is said to be malignant. It can cause death.

At this time, it is not possible to detect if a cancer is completely contained in a tumor or if a cell or two has traveled to another site. That is why chemotherapy may be suggested after a lumpectomy or mastectomy. This treatment is a safety factor to prevent the cancer cells from growing elsewhere in the body.

There are over 100 types of cancer. Certain types of cancer cells grow in the breast. Different kinds grow in the ovaries. In order for a physician to effectively treat cancer, it is important that the exact kind of cancer be detected.

To determine this information, a sample of the tumor is needed. A needle aspiration, a needle biopsy or a surgical biopsy can obtain a sample of the tumor cells. The needle aspiration and biopsy can be done with a needle and syringe. Removal of the whole tumor requires an incision. The tissue sample is sent to the lab to determine the type of cell.

The resulting report identifies if cancer is present and the exact type. Often a tumor is not cancer (malignant) but benign, meaning good. That would be good news all right, because a benign tumor does not spread. It just stays where it is, growing larger until it is removed.

What Is Oncology?

Physicians who specialize in the detection and treatment of cancer are called oncologists. Medical oncologists treat patients with chemicals. Surgical oncologists operate on patients to remove malignant tumors. The study of cancer is called oncology. When a definitive diagnosis of cancer is made, the oncologist determines what kinds of chemicals can best target and kill the specific type of cancer cells. Fortunately, a selection of these toxic drugs to effectively treat cancer is now available. Successful treatment means killing the cancer cells. In order to do this, toxic or poisonous drugs are needed.

What Is Chemotherapy?

Another bit of good news related to the fact that cancer cells grow faster than normal cells is that those cancer cells operate in a hyperactive state. They absorb more nutrients, more fluid, more of everything, including more of the toxic drug that will kill them. They can hardly wait to absorb the toxic drug because it is specially targeted to the specific cancer in the specific organ. That is what chemotherapy is all about.

The name itself denotes the treatment. *Chemo* means chemical or drug and *therapy* means treatment. The poisonous drug administered to the person with cancer affects every cell in the body, but it affects the cancer cells more because they absorb more of the poisonous drug. But owing to the potency of the chemicals received in the course of treatment, the person experiences certain side effects. These side effects are somewhat predictable although they occur in varying degrees. Some can be treated, some avoided and some just tolerated. For most women, the end goal makes the inconvenience of the symptoms tolerable.

CHEMOTHERAPY: The use of chemicals or drugs to treat illness, especially cancer. Anticancer agents are toxic to cells and destroy both normal and abnormal cells.

The medical oncologist determines the toxic drug or combination of toxic drugs that will be most effective in treating the kind of cancer that afflicts the person. This physician also monitors blood levels, treats symptoms and observes suppression of cellular function. Also, the medical oncologist prescribes medications to prevent and manage adverse symptoms and instructs the person on the advantages and dangers of the chemotherapy.

A Closer Look at Chemotherapy Drugs

Many anticancer drugs kill cancer cells by affecting DNA synthesis or function, but they vary in how they work within the cell cycle. Chemotherapeutic drugs can be classified as cell-cycle specific (CCS) or cell-cycle nonspecific (CCNS). CCS drugs attack cancer cells when the cells enter a certain phase of reproduction; they are most effective against rapidly growing tumors. CCNS drugs can destroy cancer cells in any phase of the cell cycle. In many situations, both CCS and CCNS drugs may be given in combination over an extended period of time to achieve the maximum effect.

What Is the Procedure
of Administering Chemotherapy?

Usually, chemotherapy is administered intravenously to persons on an outpatient basis, although there are a few chemotherapy drugs that can be taken by mouth. During the administration of intravenous drugs, the needle can be inserted into a peripheral vein in the hand or forearm. That is the route I chose for my chemotherapy.

> **PERIPHERAL VEINS:** Surface vessels that you can see.
> **INTRAVENOUS:** Means "into a vein."

Another choice is to have a central line (called a tube or port) inserted into a large vein such as the vena cava. This tube has a rubber stopper at the tip through which the needle is inserted for each chemotherapy treatment so the person's arm does not have to get stuck with a needle for each treatment and each blood draw.

> **VENA CAVA:** The largest vein in the body. It extends through the abdominal and chest cavities and returns the unoxygenated blood to the heart so the blood can be pumped to the lungs, reoxygenated and recirculated through the body.

The insertion of this port is often done during the mastectomy surgery but can be done in a short outpatient surgical procedure at any time. The needle through which the chemotherapy is administered is inserted through the rubber stopper that flows directly into the vena cava.

There are two kinds of central lines. One is called a Hickman catheter and the other is called a medaport. The tip of the Hickman catheter is placed outside the body. Special care is needed at the site so an infection does not occur. The tip of the medaport, on the other hand, is placed under the skin. So each time chemo is administered, the skin is punctured but no veins are probed.

The chemo drugs travel through all the veins of the body and are irritating to them. However, some feel that the use of a port to avoid the direct flow of the chemo into the peripheral veins helps to preserve them.

Persons with small and hard-to-find veins and those who require many doses of chemotherapy may want to consider having a port inserted. Nurses will instruct the person on port care in order to prevent infection at the site of insertion.

Receiving the Chemotherapy

So where do you go to have chemotherapy? This really depends on a number of things, including what facilities are available in your area. Facilities also vary in physical layout. To receive my treatments, I reported to an oncology clinic that contained three large rooms. All adults who were receiving chemotherapy on a certain day were together in these rooms. It was a comfortable setting. Lounge chairs were arranged around the walls with straight-backed chairs and tables for visitors.

I found that choosing just the right chair is important if you have a goal in mind. Some patients want to make a friend or find a person with whom to make conversation. Often patients bring a friend or relative along to keep them company. Some patients want to spend time alone with their thoughts so they may seek a corner

The Importance of a Blood Count

By Joanna Brell, MD

Almost all chemotherapeutic agents inhibit bone marrow function so that levels of red cells, white cells and platelets are episodically low during treatment. If a person starts a chemotherapy session with low levels of these vital cells, they will predictably encounter dangerously lower levels during the chemotherapy cycle. The oncologist may delay treatment or change the dosage to help prevent this problem. The blood counts tell us how well the bone marrow is working and must be assessed before each cycle of chemotherapy is administered.

chair with a table on either side of them. Some choose a chair far away from the nurses' station in order to enjoy a quieter zone.

The chemo receiver is instructed to eat something light before arriving. During the treatment, crackers, juice, coffee and tea may be available.

I had my blood drawn by a phlebotomist on arrival at the clinic. My oncologist then evaluated the results of the blood work to be sure the levels of red and white cells were appropriate. Before administering the chemo, my oncologist talked to me about what to expect with this treatment, conveyed special instructions and answered any questions.

The oncology nurses were very friendly and helpful. I found them to be an invaluable source of information. They informed me of side effects that might occur, answered my questions and suggested methods of tempering the effects of the chemo.

After reviewing the blood test results, the oncologist orders the dosages of the specific drugs then the onsite pharmacist mixes the chemotherapy solution and gives it to an oncology nurse to administer. There are usually two drugs given intravenously before the chemotherapy solution begins.

First is an antiemetic drug that eliminates or minimizes nausea. Although not all patients experience nausea, this drug is given as a precaution. If nausea occurs, it usually does not occur until several hours after the chemotherapy is completed, perhaps the evening after a morning administration. Many patients drive themselves to and from therapy without mishap.

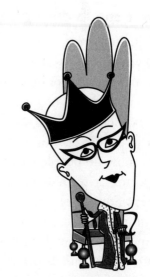

Picking just the right chair was important to achieving certain goals.

The second drug is a steroid to lessen the body's reaction to the toxic chemotherapy drug. After the administration of those drugs is completed, it is time for the chemotherapy.

Receiving intravenous chemotherapy should not be a painful event. If the patient experiences a burning feeling within the peripheral vein as the medication is given, the nurse should be notified so the rate of administration can be slowed. This burning sensation would not occur if the drugs were delivered directly into the vena cava through the port. Occasionally, a headache might develop during administration. If that occurs, the nurse would slow the rate of administration.

The actual administration of all drugs takes between 2 and 5 hours, depending on the drug and the person's tolerance to it. The total time of the visit may be longer because of meeting with the oncologist and the lab work.

During the course of administration, a patient may want to walk to the bathroom or to the refrigerator. The intravenous medication bags are hung on a portable pole with wheels to facilitate mobility.

What to Do during the Chemotherapy Administration

Chemotherapy is administered to persons with many kinds of malignant diseases. In my case, we all shared the same treatment room so there were men and women present who had had various types of surgeries or no surgery. Children scheduled to receive chemotherapy were treated in a separate area from adults. Not all cancer centers administer chemotherapy to children.

So how do people pass the hours in this room? Some choose this opportunity to share symptoms, happy moments and miseries with others. Some look forward to this meeting to see how life has treated others who receive their treatments on the same day. They have formed an informal support group.

Others recipients prefer to avail themselves of some quiet time. They prefer to nap or read. They seem to be able to tune out those who are sharing all manner of information.

Some choose to use this time to compile a journal of their thoughts and experiences about this time in their lives. Some write letters or copy recipes for future meals.

I decided that this would be a good time to read a book. I recognized at the outset that for me, it had to be a book with a light plot and perhaps a little romance. It was hard for me to concentrate on anything of much substance because of all the activity in the room. It turned out that I spent much of my time eavesdropping. Being nosy paid off, and I actually learned a lot! I listened to the nurses as they instructed other patients, explained various procedures and answered questions. I found it to be quite enlightening.

A professional friend of mine who also had breast cancer planned to listen to classical music or a book on tape during her treatment. She brought her Walkman and tuned into Mozart. But the environment proved to be too confusing to concentrate on the music. So the next time, she brought a book on tape. Again, between the interruptions of the staff with educational messages and the physician with other points of discussion, she was unable to concentrate on the story line. But she was determined to block out those voices in the surrounding group that were discussing various experiences about vomiting and having attacks of diarrhea. That was more than she wanted to know. So for the succeeding treatments, she brought only the earphones and left the Walkman at home. She lightened her load and succeeded in attaining her goal.

Cycle of Administration

Each anticancer drug has an optimal cycle of administration. For example, for maximum effectiveness, it may be administered once every three weeks for a total of four treatments. In some cases, if the symptoms are more severe than the person is able to tolerate, the oncologist may decrease the concentration of the chemotherapy. In that instance, therapy may be extended in order to kill all of the cancer cells.

Certain types of cancer cells require more than one type of chemotherapy administered sequentially. Also, more than one cycle of chemotherapy may be necessary if the cancer has spread to other organs before the original site has been detected and treated. Cancer that has already metastasized is not in its earliest stages. This cancer may not be curable but may be arrested at its current level. With repeated cycles of chemotherapy, this cancer may be controlled.

What Causes Cancer?

The actual cause of cancer is not known. Theories abound. Many factors are called carcinogens. That means those items that may influence cells to turn into cancer and begin to grow unchecked. There are some definite carcinogenic links such as smoking and lung cancer. No definite cause has been identified for breast cancer.

Family history seems to influence the development of cancer. That is, those persons with a family history of cancer of a particular organ may have a greater chance of developing the same kind of cancer. Those persons are wise to remind the physician of this family history at their annual physical exam so that the particular organ can be thoroughly checked.

MY MEDICAL TEAM MEMBERS

BREAST SURGEON: Removes the lump or tumor, inserts drains to prevent swelling and follows the recovery from the initial operation to healing. Performs follow-up exams for a period of two years after the initial surgery to ensure no reccurrence has developed. This schedule depends on the individual physician.

PLASTIC OR RECONSTRUCTIVE SURGEON: A surgeon who implants prostheses or rebuilds the breast with muscle and fat from the abdominal wall, back or buttock. Follow-up visits depend on the type of surgery and the physician.

ONCOLOGIST: A medical doctor who prescribes the most effective treatment for the type of malignant growth and follows the person through this therapy and beyond.

ONCOLOGY NURSE: A registered nurse (RN) who is specially schooled and certified to administer anticancer drugs and counsel persons about self-care during treatment.

CLINICAL NURSE SPECIALIST IN ONCOLOGY: An RN with a master's degree who specializes in the physical exam, counseling and meeting with groups of persons undergoing treatment for a malignant disease.

Certain cancers are known to metastasize to certain organs. Breast cancer commonly metastasizes to the liver, lungs and bones, although it can also invade the brain. After developing and treating breast cancer, the liver and lungs are regularly observed to be sure that no metastasis ("mets") have occurred. If bones are affected, the usual indicator is pain.

Used individually or in combination, anticancer drugs can "cure" those breast cancers that are detected in the early stages following surgical removal. These drugs travel through the body to find any stray cancer cells and kill them. In later stages, these drugs slow the growth of the cancer thereby lengthening the life of the afflicted person.

Reconstructive Surgery

The mastectomy is usually performed before chemotherapy is administered. I needed to decide whether or not to have reconstructive surgery after my breast was removed. That is, I wanted to decide if I planned to have a prosthesis permanently implanted to replace the breast that was removed. For me, the alternative was to leave the chest wall flat and wear a bra with silicone breast prosthesis in the cup to mimic the missing breast.

The decision of having reconstruction surgery does not need to be made before the mastectomy. This decision can be made anytime after the breast is removed. However, the later decision necessitates another trip to the operating room and I wanted to keep those to a minimum.

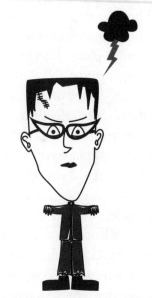

I wasn't sure what to expect after reconstructive surgery.

I gave these choices some serious thought and decided to have the reconstructive surgery. Of course, the bra with the silicone prosthesis is supposed to stay in place. But I could picture myself reaching up for something with the arm on the mastectomy side and having the silicone prosthesis riding up to my shoulder. I had enough trouble keeping my bra in place before the mastectomy. So I didn't think that I'd have any luck with only one breast to anchor it. So I opted for the reconstructive surgery.

I had no real knowledge of how the reconstructive procedure was performed. I assumed that the breast prosthesis would be placed in the cavity that remained after removal of the breast tissue. I assumed it would take one trip to the operating room. I assumed wrong on both counts.

I mentioned my simple theory to the plastic surgeon who was going to perform the procedure. As I watched the smoke pour out of his ears, I was thankful that he didn't have a scalpel in his hand! He informed me that he studied for years to learn to perform this procedure and indicated that the operation was more complex than I had thought.

It turned out that my reconstructive surgery necessitated two trips to the operating room. During the first trip, the breast surgeon removed the cancerous breast tissue. Then the plastic surgeon came along and separated the chest muscle from the chest wall. The next step was to place an inflatable breast prosthesis called a tissue expander between the chest wall and the muscle where it was sewn in place. This prosthesis contained a little saline and a rubber stopper under the skin through which more saline would be added.

Every three or four weeks, I returned to the physician's office where more saline was added until the chest muscle was overstretched. This was done so that the chest muscle wouldn't contract back into place when the permanent prosthesis was put in place—so it matched the opposite breast.

When enough saline had been added to overstretch the chest muscle, I looked like I was carrying a cantaloupe in my bra. And I had to live with that look for about seven weeks. This whole inflation process took place over several months.

Then came the second trip to surgery to have the tissue expander removed and a permanent prosthesis implanted. I had a choice of a soft, breast-shaped prosthesis containing either saline or silicone. Although the after-surgery appearance is the same, the silicone prosthesis has the weight and consistency of a natural breast whereas the saline-filled prosthesis is lighter weight and does not have a breast-like consistency. I chose the saline prosthesis. I learned that if I chose the silicone prosthesis I would need to participate in an ongoing study to be sure the silicone wasn't seeping out and traveling around my body.

In some hospitals, the implant technique involves inserting one saline prosthesis, then overinflating it over a period of time, then decreasing the amount of fluid in that same prosthesis to match the opposite breast. That procedure involves only one trip to the operating room for reconstructive surgery.

I did not think about having chemotherapy after the lumpectomy was performed. I didn't even talk it over with my surgeon or oncologist. Because cancer spreads through the lymph system and there were no cancer cells present in my lymph nodes, I just presumed that all my cancer cells had been removed. I was happy as a lark and thought the cancer problem was resolved. I should have at least inquired about it. I did the estrogen antagonist, tamoxifen, but it wasn't effective in depressing the growth of my cancer.

After the cancer recurred and I had the mastectomy plus the reconstructive surgery, I finally started chemotherapy. I waited until the incision from the final surgery had healed before I began. What an adventure that was going to be.

Another Type of Reconstructive Surgery

Breast reconstruction involving tissue flaps from another part of the body to the chest area is another option. This means that a flap of skin, muscle and fat from the back, lower abdomen or buttocks is used to create a breast shape. This is a major operation and results in large surgical wounds and more than one trip to the operating room. Success depends on good blood supply to the flap tissue.

This type of surgery is more involved than what I had and is not always successful. The flap tissue in the breast area may not survive the transplant because of infection and poor wound healing. But it is an option that definitely should be discussed with a plastic surgeon before decisions are made.

Introduction to Postchemotherapy Symptoms

Chemicals that are administered to fight cancer affect every cell of the body. For that reason, persons receiving those toxic drugs may experience side effects. These side effects are minimized by certain medications given at the time the chemotherapy is administered. These prechemo medications vary with the type of chemo drug. In addition, some medications are ordered by the physician to be taken "as needed" over the course of treatment to make unpleasant symptoms tolerable.

Most persons receiving chemotherapy commonly experience specific symptoms. However, not every person experiences every symptom. Also, the severity of the symptoms varies. Side effects differ according to the type of chemo, the dosage and the frequency of administration. In addition, a person's physical condition at the time of treatment affects the overall tolerance.

Some factors to consider when the body begins to react to the chemo drugs are

- Some symptoms will be minor. They cause little discomfort and little disruption to daily life.

- Some symptoms will be major. They can cause much discomfort and much disruption to daily life.

- Almost all symptoms will be transient and will not last. Those that do occur are usually present during and immediately following the course of treatment.

- If severe symptoms occur and persist, the physician should be notified. Many can be relieved or muted by medication.

In the following section, symptoms associated with the aftermath of receiving chemotherapy are presented. I personally experienced most of them, but some were shared by friends. The trick was to discover how to mute them, eliminate them or prevent them from happening. This project took some research, consulting with professionals and pooling fellow patients' resources and experiences. It proved to be a challenging and rewarding project.

I found that many symptoms led me to my bathroom. In fact, I spent quite a lot of time there and became rather fond of it. That experience inspired the following poem:

If you should ask, "What's my most frequented room?"
I would probably reply, "It's my bathroom."
I spend so much of my day there, you see
Taking care of nature, goodness me.

My bodily functions were of no concern
But now with this chemo, I've taken a turn.
I keep track of secretions and excretions too
I record all this while I stay in the loo.

2

Keeping Up Appearances

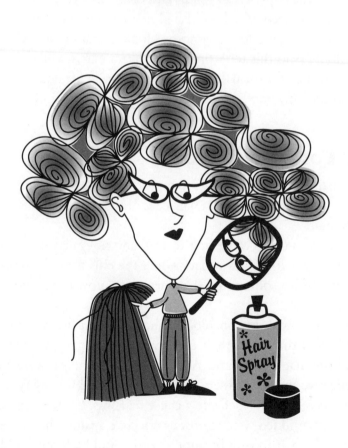

Look good, feel good. How often have you heard that axiom? It may be difficult to meet either one of those goals when you are undergoing chemotherapy.

On days when I didn't feel up to snuff, I'd try not to look in the mirror. That helped a lot. I just avoided the issue of appearance, especially when I was wearing some monstrosity to keep my bald head warm. On other days, I could look in the mirror, laugh at myself and be thankful that I would not look like this forever.

But I am a proud person who wants to look as good as I can when I leave my bathroom in the morning. On days when I was scheduled to leave my home, trying to look good was a major project. I had purchased many potions, powders and creams to disguise dark circles, make my cheeks pink and color my eyelids. It was a wonder anyone recognized me. I had never made such an effort before. I wasn't going for a glamorous look, just a moderately healthy look. And this took time. I felt like an artist with a blank canvas, but the effort usually paid off. At least my friends and relatives told me how good I looked. And I did not question their honesty.

Hair Loss: Bald Beauty

The goal of chemotherapy is to attack the fastest growing cells in the body, the cancer cells. But hair cells grow fast too. Thus, there goes the hair!

Some chemo drugs cause hair to thin and not fall out completely. Either way hair will grow back when the effects of chemotherapy are over. With some drugs, hair begins to grow back before the end of therapy.

When I met with my oncologist, she explained the various chemotherapy drugs and their effectiveness then gave me a choice. She told me that at this time, Adriamycin and cytoxen were a bit more effective than the others she had mentioned for my type of breast cancer. But they definitely cause hair loss. Some of the other drugs she mentioned were almost as effective against the cancer and cause the hair to thin but not all of it would fall out. So I thought about the choices, but not for long. I decided that I wanted to go for the "cure". I accepted the Adriamycin and cytoxen and the hair loss plan. And sure enough, I became the Bald Beauty of my neighborhood.

I was told that with my kind of chemo, hair usually begins to fall out at the end of the third week following the first treatment. And exactly on schedule, my hair came out by the handful by the third week. As I ran my fingers through my hair, I'd pinch them together and came away with a fist full of hair.

A person doesn't just wake up one morning bald as a billiard ball, Sweet Pea or Yul Brynner. Hair falls out gradually over a week or more. Some chemo patients help it along. I thought about those days when I felt like tearing my hair out. Well, now I had my chance!

When hair begins to fall out, it is everywhere. I found that it was easier to pull out the loose hair rather than to clean it up every day. If loose hair is pulled out, it doesn't land all over everything. At first, I chose not to help it along. So it fell out in the sink, on the kitchen counter, on the table, on the floor, in my food, in my bed and all over my clothes. And I ended up picking up one hair at a time throughout the house.

To decrease the amount of hair on my bed pillow in the morning, I used a satin pillowcase. There seems to be less friction between the head and a satin pillowcase than between the head and a cotton pillowcase. I learned this as I tried to maintain a hair-sprayed set after a session at the beauty salon. When I used a cotton pillow-

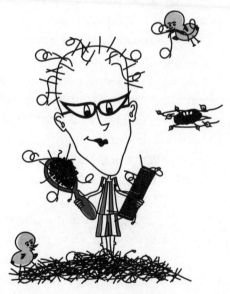

Previous bad hair days didn't seem so bad now!

case, I'd awaken in the morning looking much like a cone head, with my hair all munched up toward the top of my head. It was my beautician who recommended a satin pillowcase so my hair would slide in its proper place without sticking to the pillowcase and rearranging itself upward on my head. Thus, the hair I was about to lose didn't stick to the satin pillowcase either.

As my hair came out, it was hard to avoid feeling sad. I had to tell myself that this is a small price to pay for "the cure." I tried to disown that hair in the trash basket by thinking, "This doesn't belong to me anymore. It belongs to chemotherapy. And I don't want it!" But it did feel strange to see a part of myself, my "crowning glory," in the trash basket.

I remembered back to those days when I thought, "I hate my hair!" I had to laugh at myself because, in fact, I wanted whatever kind of hair I used to have back on my head. I had to keep reminding myself that this was a temporary state of affairs—that my lovely locks would grow back! Meanwhile the title of Miss Bald Beauty was perfect for me.

There was a time when wearing an ice cap on the head during the administration of chemo was supposed to decrease or eliminate hair loss. The reasoning behind this was that cold would constrict blood vessels in the scalp and less chemo would circulate to that site so hair follicles would not be affected. Good thought! But it didn't work because the anticancer chemicals work over a period of days, not just when administered.

Some women are left with a little fringe around the face. These hairs may be left in place and arranged so they peek out from beneath a turban, giving the illusion that there is more hair under there. Some women shave those few hairs so they are totally bald and can see at a glance when hair begins to grow. Fringe hairs left in place help to keep the head warm. Total baldness allows a lot of body heat to escape through the head.

Those fringe hairs do not grow. They become dry and brittle and eventually break off. But they can be used while they're there. They may even last until new hair grows in and then trimmed as the new hair catches up.

The Emotional Side of Hair Loss

By Barbara Tripp, RN

Women experience many different emotions while anticipating and dealing with the loss of their hair. Personal appearance and self-image go hand in hand. For some it will be no big deal. Others may contemplate or actually decline chemotherapy owing to the antici-pated trauma of losing their hair. Some shave their head before the first strand is lost, hoping to maintain a sense of control, and others hold on to each sprig of hair, even if it is "the world's worst comb-over" (a joke one woman made when discussing her own hair loss).

There is no right way or wrong way to feel, and an outsider's opin-ion of "it's just hair" can be quite hurtful. A bad hair day can stress even the most self-confident woman. When the impact is minimized the woman may believe her feelings are wrong, bad or abnormal. The lines of communication and support may break down. Identifying, acknowledging then working with and through these feelings can actually prove to be an empowering experience.

Head Coverings

Some women wear a sleep cap to bed. This is a light cotton tur-ban-type hat worn for appearance and to prevent heat loss. If this falls off during the night, the bed sheet can be tucked around the head for warmth. Use of a contour pillow helps prevent heat loss because the head sinks into it and is partially enveloped by it.

There are many head coverings available on the market. Scarves, turbans, hats and wigs can be purchased at stores or through cata-logs. Information about obtaining catalogs is located at the end of this book.

For myself, I found that the lightest and warmest head covering was the green cap that a person wears to surgery to prevent hair from falling out in the operating room. These green caps are incomparably ugly, but with two of them, one on top of the other, and a little soft stuffing in the front to give a little lift to the look, they were the perfect head covering for me. They look like the old-fashioned bowl covers that those of us of a certain age will recall from childhood. But they do the trick and keep the head warm.

Wigs

In the case of baldness, a wig can make the woman—or at least partly make the woman. It makes all the difference in the world to feel comfortable and appropriately appointed. That can happen if you think that your wig looks good on you, if it is your style and color.

I feel that it's worth taking the time and making the effort to shop until you find one that's almost you. It will never be your own hair, but hopefully you will feel comfortable in it.

Of course, some women wear wigs all the time for various reasons. Some have thin hair and some have severely receding hairlines. Whatever the reason, wigs are popular. It is a big business and the quality is improving every day.

Some women don't wear wigs after losing their hair. They may wear a scarf or a hat on their head or no head covering at all.

Wig wearing is an experience in itself. At first the wearer may feel uncomfortable, self-conscious and think that everyone is looking at her. I needed to get used to wearing my wig and to the feeling that it was not always askew—although sometimes it was.

Many wigs are quite natural looking. Some wigs are wavy and some are straight. Some are made of real human hair or a blend of human and synthetic hair. Most wigs are made of synthetic hair and their color is

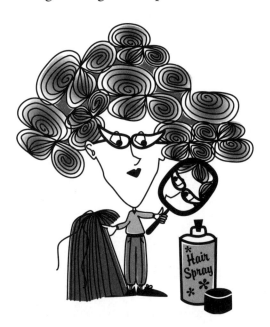

What looked good on Dolly Parton did not look good on me!

permanent. Like other synthetics, they don't fade in sunlight or after many shampoos, so order the color you want to wear.

If the wearer acts like the wig is her own hair, most people will never know. Of course, tugging on it and rearranging it in public is a dead giveaway.

Wig Shopping

I was determined to look as natural as possible for my own satisfaction. So I knew that the right wig would be important to me.

My first (and last) wig-shopping trip was a total disaster! I made an appointment at a local beauty salon that was on the list of wig-selling shops given to me by my oncologist. A beautician who was totally caught up in her migraine headache and her morning coffee met me there. She smoked her head off while she complimented me on buying a wig from a local retailer. She said that she would style it and shampoo it for me free of charge if I purchased the wig in her shop.

We went together into the back room where she had a variety of wigs. Unfortunately, they were all in boxes so I couldn't see them. Thus, I could not truly shop for a wig. I had to rely on whatever she pulled out of the boxes. I soon learned that her opinion as to what would be best for me did not agree with mine.

The first thing she did was hand me a nylon stocking cap. I was to place it over my own hair for reasons of hygiene and so wigs could be slipped on and off more easily. Because I was used to a fluffy bouffant hairdo with bangs, this skullcap resulted in a most disturbing appearance. I suddenly realized that this is what I would look like without any hair! An appalling thought!

The next thing she did was to fit three wigs on my head, one at a time, talking all the while about all the hairless women she had worked with and how wonderful she had made them look. But I looked absolutely ridiculous with those huge mounds of hair on my head! What looked good on Dolly Parton did not look good on me.

Because I thought that wig wearing would only be necessary for a few months (it turned out to be many months), I was not planning to invest the family fortune to acquire one. But I would not have hit a bison in the behind with any one of those that she put on my head that cost less than $325, plus tax! In fact, she wouldn't show me any wigs for less than $200, explaining that her husband had walked out on her and she had a child she wanted to send through college. She went on and on about how it was not her goal to gouge the public, but that she had to consider her own financial status and her right to a fair return for her services.

The conversation was so far afield from anything that concerned me at that moment, I found it absolutely ludicrous! Where was the psychology here, I wondered. The anticipation of baldness is so traumatic for a woman and as a wig seller she should have known that and approached me differently. Between the conversation and my state of shock at my upcoming appearance, I couldn't escape from there fast enough.

I had no idea where else I could go to shop for a wig so I consulted with friends who made some valuable suggestions. One even mailed her wig catalog to me. Once you are on the wig catalog list, you keep getting them for years—long after your hair has grown in—and they come from more than one source.

As was also suggested to me, I visited beauty salons in department stores. They had large catalogs on site that I could review. Of course, once you ordered a wig, it was yours because those catalogs do not accept returns. But it was an education. Over time, I learned that most of the same wigs pictured in the professional catalogs could be ordered at home from a mail order catalog and can be returned. Was I relieved! Good thing I started early enough to learn all this before my hair fell out. I wanted to be ready.

All in all, I purchased four wigs and returned three. Two were not the right color and one was not the right size. I kept the fourth wig and have been pleased with it. It did not look like my own hair, but it was close enough. I learned to live with it. It served the purpose. I wore it in public with some comfort, without feeling that I looked absurd, and I was grateful for that.

I have since learned that a wig is considered a prosthesis. Thus the cost of one wig may be covered by your health insurance. Just obtain a prescription signed by the physician and submit it with a copy of the receipt for your wig.

> **PROSTHESIS:** An artificial device that replaces a missing part of the body—in this case, hair.

Wig Styling and Care

One of the bonuses to wearing a wig is that you never worry about fixing a hairdo. Just slap on the wig and away you go. No more bad hair days!

When I had hair, I was a regular customer at the beauty salon for styling, trims and color applications. I was amazed at how much money I saved by wearing the wig. Even though the outlay of funds was substantial for the purchase and initial styling of the wig, I saved money in the end.

Although beauty shops sell wigs, the cost is considerably less if they are purchased through a catalog. Wherever it is purchased, a wig will look more natural if it is styled by a beautician. At first I didn't realize that a wig comes with an overabundance of hair so that it can be trimmed and styled for the wearer. Because I was unaware of that, I was quite put off by my initial appearance with an enormous head of hair. In fact, I looked like a wild woman. I finally figured it out and scheduled an appointment at my salon. I learned from reading about wig wearing that it is advisable to style a new wig before hair loss occurs so that the beautician can copy the person's usual appearance. So I did just that. My beautician warned me that she could trim some of the voluminous hair off but recommended not to cut too much in one sitting. She reminded me that wig hair does not grow back if it is cut too short.

Caring for a wig is not difficult. Catalogs sell special shampoos, conditioners and hair sprays made for wigs. A wig made of synthetic hair is easier to care for than one made with real hair because real hair can become dry and brittle without natural oils.

A Lasting Impression

One day, as I was reclining and reading without my wig, the doorbell rang. I dashed to the bedroom, whipped on my wig and appeared at the door somewhat breathless. Sure enough, the

United Parcel Service deliveryman needed my signature. As I was signing, he was staring. He looked abashed when I returned his clipboard and caught him.

As I carried the package across the room, I passed a mirror and glanced at myself. I stopped dead in my tracks and retraced my steps to the mirror. No wonder the poor deliveryman looked horrified. The sides of my wig winged out over the temples of my glasses, looking like I'd been partially scalped on both sides. And the temples of my glasses looked as though they were tucked under my scalp and attached to my skull. I'll bet he had a tale to tell about that day on the job.

My Hair Loss Story

Hair loss is the symptom that was foremost on my mind when I first consulted an oncologist. Would my hair fall out? When would that happen? How long would I be without hair? When would it begin to grow in?

My first consult was with an oncologist who was handsome, middle-aged, male and bald. Hair was the last thing on his mind but the first thing on mine. My questions must have seemed frivolous to him. He was ready to explain many of the statistics about recurrence and "cure" and I was primarily interested in information about my hair!

During this preliminary visit before surgery, he told me that I wouldn't necessarily lose my hair. I was so relieved! I clung to that belief. I thought I could take anything if I didn't lose my hair! It may not have been the most stylish do in the world but it was the only do I had. My anxiety lowered and my hope was restored. I felt that I could handle any situation now.

My second visit with him occurred after the mastectomy. During that meeting he told me that I probably would lose my hair. I was stunned! To think that he had told me otherwise really bothered me. Of course, he added that he couldn't give me a definite answer until he saw my pathology report. Then he would know exactly which chemicals would be most effective. That decision would tell the tale about my precious hair. I wish he had explained that to me at my first visit. I would have been better prepared for the possibility of losing my hair.

Now I was unsure if I wanted this physician as my oncologist. I wanted to completely rely on and trust the oncologist I chose. As a type A personality, I needed definite answers to definite questions. I understood the words "I don't know" and "I'm not sure." But I needed to know as exactly as possible what would happen to me.

So I sought another opinion and was glad that I did. I went to a lovely, young, female oncologist who was trained at a medical center and who happened to have lots of hair and did lots of interesting things with it. I just knew she would understand that a cancer "cure" was important to me but my hair was a major concern to me as well.

Another Hair Loss Story

My 38-year-old niece and namesake, Maureen, explained to her husband and three small children that the medication she would take to treat her cancer would cause her hair to fall out. However, instead of allowing the cancer to cause her baldness, she planned to take control of the situation and have her head shaved. In preparation for this event, she needed to order a wig.

So she and her 2-year-old daughter, Carolyn, sat on the sofa every evening for a week leafing through catalogs to select the wig and the color of hair that would look the most natural. Carolyn took great pride in being a part of this important process and took it very seriously.

Eventually, the day came when Maureen's head was to be shaved. She and a girlfriend made arrangements at Maureen's beauty salon to go in one hour before the shop opened. They brought coffee and sweet rolls and tried to make a celebration of it. Another step toward the cancer "cure".

The group decided to have the sides and back of Maureen's head shaved but to leave a short growth on the top, like a brush cut or military cut. This would be enough of a shock for the family to get used to.

Maureen carefully gathered her hair from the floor and took it home to Carolyn. There, she and Carolyn put it in a box and laid it in the backyard so the birds would find it and use it to make their nests. Carolyn reported this to every visitor who arrived to visit that week. Proudly, she told each one that her mom's hair was going to make the birds' nests soft and warm for the baby birds. That helped shift the focus from Maureen's hairstyle and gave a purpose to the shaved hair.

Where Have My Eyebrows Gone?

Loss of facial hair also occurs with chemotherapy. This results in a denuded appearance. Without facial hair, the skin appears like the skin on a nectarine rather than the skin on a peach.

Body hair is lost as well. That may include eyebrows and eyelashes. It definitely includes leg and underarm hair. The good news is that shaving legs and underarms will not be needed while the chemo is working. Sometimes pubic hair is lost too. So far, no wigs are available for that location.

After my third dose of chemo, I realized that my eyebrows and lashes were gone. Mascara was out, but eyebrows were certainly a necessity. When I applied my face makeup, I tried to remember where my eyebrows had been so I could pencil them appropriately. How close to the nose did they begin? How high should they be drawn? Where was the arch located? Where did they begin to descend? These were important questions to me because I didn't want two question-mark-type eyebrows drawn on my face.

Eventually, I figured out that my eyebrow line was located behind the top edge of my eyeglasses. This served as a benchmark for me. Of course, I had to take my glasses off to put my eyebrows on so I still had to remember where they began, arched and ended. And although I was concerned that they be in the right place, I realized that my brows couldn't be seen very well behind my glasses when I wore them. I was thankful for that.

Another defining line had disappeared! No hair, no hairline. I tried to apply base makeup only on my face, not on my scalp. I figured out where I thought my hairline had been and where I thought the wig would sit but overshot that with the first few applications so my wig got smeared with some base makeup on the underside. Eventually, I got the knack of it.

Makeupless: Another Approach

Each time I went to the oncology center for another chemo treatment, I noticed that there were women there who were hairless like myself but wore no makeup. They appeared in their pure feminine form without any false aids. I got to thinking about that.

I never leave home without full face makeup in place. I think I could seriously scare someone in my natural state, so these women fascinated me.

As I thought about their looks, I realized that there was a loveliness to it. They were comfortable with themselves in this sleek and guileless state. They looked proud and almost regal, like the vestal virgins of Rome. I was proud of them and a little envious of their strength of character. I was not at all so secure in myself that I would go out unadorned, without my face makeup and my wig. I put it all on even to go to chemotherapy sessions. In fact, I even went to surgery with my face makeup on although I did have to remove my nail polish. So I have given lots of thought to the natural look. I've decided that I like it. It's so honest, pure and feminine.

New Hair

Usually, a wig is worn only until the real hair returns. That takes longer than I thought. Because hair only grows about 1/2 inch per month, there are many months between the initial stubble and a pageboy. Likewise, it will be many months before it's worthwhile to fire up the curling iron.

Fortunately, hair loss resulting from chemotherapy is not a permanent condition. New hair growth can be seen in 5 to 6 weeks after the last treatment. Of course, it may grow in a different color or it may be curly instead if it was previously straight. That is the adventurous part of new hair growth. Some women retain their wigs until they can get control of whatever grows in and for future bad hair days.

When new hair begins to grow, wearing the wig or turban all the time should be avoided. New hair is fragile and will break off with constant rubbing. Those unflattering caps that are worn to the operating room are especially good to wear at this time. Although the wearer may look like a French baker, these caps hold body heat in and don't rub against the hair.

If coloring is desired, the use of a rinse rather than a permanent dye is suggested. The rinse only coats the delicate hairs, whereas dye penetrates them, making them porous and breakable. It's safer to wait until the hair becomes longer and stronger to use hair dye.

Hoping for Stubble

Every morning beginning in the fourth week after my final treatment, I'd run my hand over my leg, from ankle to knee, to see if any hair was growing on my head. I'd rubbed my legs instead of my head because I didn't want to wear out the new hair on my head in case there was some there. I'd hoped for stubble. But day after day, week after week, I'd find the skin smooth as silk. Most of my life I had hoped there would be no stubble, but times had changed. I figured that when the hair follicles reactivated themselves, all my hair would begin to grow at the same time—legs, underarms and head. I was ready for hair!

Because my beautician had told me that hair grows at the rate of 1/2 inch per month, I realized why it took so long to see any hair up there. The first month consisted of hair growth within the hair follicle! I could see that it would be a long time before I could return to my hair salon for help.

To my surprise, the hair on my head grew before the hair on my legs and underarms did. Sure enough, at the beginning of the sixth week after my last chemo administration, the tiniest hairs began to peek out of the hair follicles on my scalp. Fine and soft like the hair on a newborn baby, there was too little of it to guess the color. At the beginning of the seventh week, I had a quarter inch growth on my head. Now it was beginning to show but the quality began to change.

The first quarter inch of my new hair was soft and feathery. But as it grew it became bristly and kinky curly. Oh my goodness. I hated to complain because it was hair and it kept my head warm, but it was very unlike any hair I had ever had before!

Another quarter inch and I felt like a human ChiaPet! Each kinky hair stood straight out from its hair follicle. There was no controlling it, and it felt like steel wool. As the hair grew, it became straight and very coarse—like a grizzly bear's hair. This was some experience!

Of course, the color was problematic as well. I had white hair on the sides, salt and pepper on top and dark in back. Miss Clairol, here I come!

So off to the health food store I went to find some herb or chemical to encourage hair growth. There I purchased Super Biotin 2500 mcg capsules, a dietary supplement. No claims are made that guarantee hair growth and the Food and Drug Administration has not evaluated Biotin for this. But I was ready to try anything. After 12 weeks, I had little more than 1/2 inch on the top and sides of my head.

I noticed that after a couple of weeks of taking Biotin, my facial hair was longer than the hair on my head. I couldn't believe it! On a routine visit to my medical doctor, I told him of the situation and asked what I should do. He said that I should stay out of the health food store. Big help!

The next step was to remove those facial hairs. I was beginning to look like Father Time. I purchased Surgi-Cream to cream away unwanted facial hair. I had to be careful on my cheeks, because I didn't want to cream away the head hair in front of my ears. Where did my facial hair end and my head hair begin? I didn't want sideburns but I didn't want to remove more hair than I needed to either. I had so little hair on my head that I valued every one. What a dilemma. I finally applied the cream and it turned out OK. I left more sideburns than was necessary and I missed a spot on my left jaw, but I removed most of the facial hair and left my head hair in place. I was glad when that was over. Then it was time to tackle the problem of color.

Hair Color

I decided to apply a honey brown rinse. At least with some color, it would look like I had more hair. I forgot that even temporary hair dye colors everything it touches. It colored my blouse, my forehead, my ears and my scalp. Actually, my scalp took the color better than did my hair.

The white hair on the sides turned out blond, the top and back turned out dark brown and my scalp, ears, face and blouse turned out black. So I repeated the process the next day, hoping that the hair would take more color and I could shampoo the color off my scalp, ears and face without losing all the color on my hair. Nothing is as easy as it sounds!

In a few days, I returned to the store and bought a darker brown for the sides of my hair and a solution to remove the color from my face and ears. The saleswoman couldn't believe that my scalp took so much color. She said that the color usually comes off the scalp and skin when rinsing with water. But with my scalp colored, it looked like I had more hair.

The second shade took more evenly and I wore it for a few days. Then I noticed that the hair above my ears had turned pink! I hadn't realized that the metal temples of my glasses reacted to the rinse and turned whatever hair it contacted to a shade of pink. Oh well. Again, I headed back to the store still wearing my wig.

After my third visit to purchase a darker shade, the saleslady suggested that I give up this project, go to a salon and have it professionally dyed with permanent color. Gee. And I was such a good customer!

In the ninth week after my last chemo treatment, I noticed that in addition to having hair on my head, my nose hair and pubic hairs were sprouting. I was beginning to feel like myself again.

Eventually, the quality of my locks returned to their normal silky straight self and I have been thankful ever since. But what an evolution took place on my head.

> *Pansies are purple, violets are blue,*
> *Whatever happened to my hairdo?*
> *Oh, there it is in the trash,*
> *It all fell out in a flash.*
> *I know someday my locks will grow*
> *And I'll be ready, that I know.*
> *Some days the cost of "cure" seems big*
> *Thank goodness I can wear my wig.*

Attire

"Clothes make the woman" is an axiom that has been heard for years. The way clothes hang on a person is an important factor in appearance.

Without question, clothes hang differently when one breast is missing or when one surgical appliance (tissue expander) is overinflated to the size of half a cantaloupe during the process of breast reconstruction. Whatever the reason, symmetry is a factor that relates to the way clothes look on a woman.

Of course, symmetry is available through surgical reconstruction as well as with prosthesis fitted into a brassiere. But those are not options until the healing time between the mastectomy and reconstruction is complete. Camouflaging the physique before that time is an important consideration.

I found that bulk and wearing a separate top and bottom to be the answer for me. Separates allow a blousing of the top that can distract attention from thoughts of what's underneath.

It is difficult, uncomfortable and perhaps painful to wear a regular bra until months after the mastectomy and until the reconstruction incision has healed. Wearing a tee shirt under a blouse adds enough bulk to camouflage the shape.

Wearing a jacket over two layers of tops helps, too. A loose-fitting sweater that buttons at the waist and blouses over the chest works well also.

In addition, loose-fitting clothes help disguise weight gain to some degree. Some women gain weight because of what and how much they eat and some do because of fluid retention. I found that wearing a relaxed style of clothing such as sweatpants and large blouses to be comfortable.

A Fashion Challenge

I was fortunate to have my surgery in the fall so that layering clothes during the winter months added to my comfort. It might have been a different story, however, in the summer months. With all those layers I might have had to sit in front of an air conditioner or use one of those handheld, battery-operated fans.

During reconstruction, I was quite uncomfortable with the over-inflated tissue expander that helped stretch my chest muscle in preparation for the permanent implant. I found it impossible to move my arm toward the center of my body because of this huge melon-like object attached to my chest. The other side was small, so I looked lopsided and off balance. During my cantaloupe interlude, people who didn't know me thought I was a buxom woman who had survived a mastectomy on the opposite side of the actual operative site. So the more I camouflaged my chest, the fewer questions I had to answer.

Dry Skin: Alligator Hide

The fact that many glands stop working or function very little during chemotherapy was one side effect that took me completely by surprise. The cause of this glandular suppression is unknown to the medical community. For example, there is little saliva, no perspiration and no oil gland secretion. All glands are affected.

Without oil gland secretion, the entire body's skin becomes dry. To prevent the "alligator hide look," lotion should be applied frequently. Prolonged hot tub baths and harsh soaps encourage drying so they should be avoided.

Frequent handwashing is important to prevent colds and infections. After handwashing, an alcohol-free hand lotion can be applied to avoid dry skin. If hands become extremely dry, the skin cracks open and bleeds. This condition is hard to heal and also is a hazard because an opening in the skin is an entry point for infection-causing bacteria. Alcohol-free lotions often come in a tube rather than in a pump bottle because they are creamier and more solid. Some brands to consider are the body creams and hand creams from Bath & Body Works. Among other brands are Keri lotion, Mary Kay and Lubriderm. The label on each container lists ingredients so the presence of alcohol can be detected.

During chemotherapy when oil-producing glands are suppressed, hands should be protected from harsh chemicals and harsh detergents. Kitchen gloves can be worn when washing dishes and floors. Antibacterial hand soap can be used for handwashing, but hand sanitizers like Purell are drying to the skin.

My Story

Shortly after treatments began, I was particularly aware of the dry skin on my hands. I was fearful of the skin cracking open and increasing my vulnerability to infection, so on one of my mall walks, I visited a lotion shop and asked for suggestions.

The clerk told me about cotton stretch gloves. She suggested that I liberally apply baby oil, alcohol-free lotion or cream to my hands at bedtime then wear the gloves all night. What a treat for my thirsty skin! My hands were well conditioned by morning.

Another facet of the lack of oil gland secretion was that my face lost its oily quality, so one application of makeup looked as fresh in the evening as it did when first applied in the morning. The same application could serve for days because it didn't change. It never looked oily or smeared.

I didn't perspire during chemotherapy either. So during a hot flash, I would whip off my wig for heat to escape but no perspiration was available to help me cool off. Of course, there was no underarm odor either. A mixed blessing.

At the conclusion of treatments, my glands began to function again. The first glands to wake up were the sweat glands on my scalp. So when a hot flash would strike, perspiration ran off my scalp, but my underarms and forehead were dry. What a weird way of cooling off!

It was two months after my last treatment that my oil and sweat glands began to function normally. That was a big help in cooling off, but I had to find my deodorant once again.

> *Where, oh where, has my soft skin gone?*
> *And why is my skin so dry?*
> *Why have my oil glands retired?*
> *When lubrication is required.*
> *I'm using lotion by the gallon*
> *My skin is well oiled with lanolin.*

I hope this restores my lovely skin
Before I slip and bang my shin.

Brittle Nails, Rough Cuticles

My fingernails have always been my favorite feature about my appearance. I'd always been meticulous about them. I kept them filed and polished and occasionally indulged in a professional manicure. So you can imagine how distressed I was to learn that chemotherapy could cause nails to crack, split and break. I read that nails could become brittle and the cuticles dry and rough. That was bad news to me! I needed to do something about this.

I immediately sought professional help and learned that the use of a cuticle cream to lubricate and soften the skin around the nails can minimize damage. Another technique recommended to me was to push back the cuticles with other fingernails or the towel after handwashing. My oncologist warned me not to trim the cuticles because any opening in the skin can result in an infection when the white blood cell count is low.

Off I went to the store to purchase a liquid nail conditioner to nourish and strengthen my nails. I was instructed to apply this over both bare nails and polished nails because it supposedly penetrated nail polish to work its magic. I was determined to use this product every other day as directed for maximum effect.

I have always applied several layers of polish over a base coat to strengthen and protect my nails from breaking. And in recent years, I've used a nonacetone polish remover because it's less drying to the nails than an acetone-based remover. Thus, nails are less brittle.

I still needed to solve the problem of preventing nails from cracking and breaking during chemotherapy, so I launched into a new program to strengthen them.

First I turned to Jell-O. When I was a little girl, my mother told me that gelatin would make my nails strong, and I never forgot that advice. I ate so much Jell-O that my whole body jiggled like a mountain of gelatin. Although it may have helped a little, it did not take care of the nail problem. (And, by the way, my body is still jiggling.)

I decided to prevent cracks and breaks by using my nail repair routine. That is, I applied a thin coat of nail glue over the top and underside of nail edges to strengthen them, using a toothpick to spread and smooth it. I didn't realize when I first used this product that it acts like Super Glue. It dries fast and permanently sticks together any surfaces that come in contact with it! When I began my repair routine, I had only one thin letter under the glue container. In the process of applying the glue to my nails, a drop fell onto the letter. It spread instantly and stuck the letter to my lovely white Formica tabletop permanently. It took much time, elbow grease, acetone polish remover and a very sharp knife to remove that letter from my tabletop.

I have a friend who owns a nail shop in New York City. The most beautiful manicures on the most beautiful people walked out of there, so I followed her advice about nail care. She told me that when a nail split or broke, I should apply a neatly trimmed piece of an unused tea bag (minus the tea leaves) and anchor it with clear polish or nail glue. This paper contains fibers and is strong enough to hold the broken edges together. When the initial application was dry, I covered it with a coat of either clear polish or nail glue. Nail glue is harder and more protective than clear polish but it is not easy to work with.

A Nail Tale

When a friend of mine underwent chemotherapy, her nails were so broken she had acrylic nails applied. They looked beautiful on her long, thin fingers.

One day, she was especially nauseated and dashed to the bathroom. She held her wig with one hand and grasped the toilet seat with the other as she lost her lunch. When she looked up, she spotted a multiple-legged creature zipping across the floor behind the toilet. Determined that only two-legged species would inhabit her abode, she later drove to the hardware store and purchased a bug box. This product contains a Super Glue-like adhesive throughout the interior. The bug is drawn into the box by a mating scent and is trapped there with its legs stuck to the wall.

As she set up the box, she reached in to push the end wall upright and the acrylic nail of her index finger stuck to the side wall. No matter how she coaxed and maneuvered, the box would not come loose. She could hardly appear that evening at her husband's company dinner party with a roach box stuck to her index finger. So she gave a mighty tug and the acrylic nail came off her finger, but continued to stick to the box. Now what to do? She had nine beautiful fingernails and one stub without polish.

Because it was too late to dash to the nail shop, she had to polish the stubby nail and carry on. She was consumed with the thought of hiding that hand most of the evening, but although it did look odd, no one at the party made a comment.

> *Broken, brittle, cracked and chipped,*
> *What kind of a manicure is this?*
> *I want my nails to be long and pink,*
> *I want them gorgeous quick as a wink.*
> *I'll repair them, wrap them and treat them with care*
> *And then I'll be ready to go anywhere.*

Flushed Face and Neck: Tomato Face

A flushed face and neck will develop soon after treatment if it is going to occur. The face and neck appear bright red and feel hot to the touch. It is not related to a fever. Although this is not an uncommon side effect, it does not happen to everyone and may not occur after each treatment.

There is no logical explanation as to why this occurs, but it is not harmful. The redness can last up to 24 hours or a little longer. However, if a rash appears or if the skin becomes itchy, the physician should be notified.

My Facial Event

This tomato face phenomenon happened to me the morning after the third treatment. It had never happened before and never happened again.

I awoke feeling like my usual self. As I passed the bathroom mirror, I happened to glance up and saw this bright red person! I could hardly believe it! I had never read or heard about this in my entire professional life. But, luckily, during the course of my treatment the previous day, another woman was discussing this symptom with the nurse as her chemo was being administered. Had I not been there at that time and been eavesdropping, I might really have become most anxious or even panicky! It is such an unusual happening. The face and neck are completely bright red and hot to the touch but there is no fever. What an experience!

One would think that after all I had read and after all the oncologist and nurses had taught me, I would have been well versed in any event that could possibly happen. But here I was with a totally unread-about, unheard-about experience. Thank goodness for eavesdropping.

It is important and common for oncologists and nurses to try to explain every possible event that could happen and give each patient a folder with lots of printed information. But that is almost an impossible task and an unfair expectation. So if you have a question or have heard about a peculiar symptom like this one, do ask about it. You might even ask about any exceptional symptoms that could happen, thus covering most of the bases.

> *I never asked to be a Red Hot Mama,*
> *Nor did I ask to be the star in this drama.*
> *My tomato face is not a common occurrence*
> *But I think I'll consider personal fire insurance!*

Weight Gain or Loss: Plumper or Svelter

A hefty appetite and a sweet tooth are almost certain to result in weight gain. Because breast cancer often strikes in mid to late life when people have a tendency to gain weight, increasing the volume of food consumed and eating more sweets is likely to tip the scales toward heavy.

I learned that attitude plays a part. I felt that because I was a cancer survivor, I should treat myself. Because I didn't deserve cancer, I brought out the ice cream and poured on the hot fudge sauce. Later I discovered the connection between my attitude and my waistline.

Conversely, some women lose weight during the course of chemotherapy. This can occur because of nausea, vomiting and loss of appetite and prolonged diarrhea. If mouth sores are present, it may be too painful to eat. Naturally, if a person does not eat, weight loss will occur. If solid food cannot be tolerated, food supplements can be consumed to provide nutrients. The physician should be notified if severe symptoms occur. Medications to eliminate or minimize these symptoms are available.

Assuaging My Hunger

I was ravenously hungry throughout my chemotherapy. So, never one to deprive myself, I ate. I decided I'd worry about my waistline after chemotherapy when my energy level increased and my interest in exercise returned. Of course, I had never been interested in exercise, but one can hope to change old habits.

When I went to the oncologist's office for the second treatment, I had to weigh

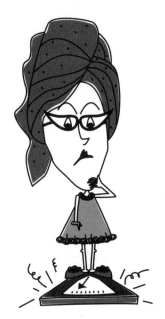

Everything was relative. Chemo increased my appetite.

Diet Changes

By Barbara Tripp, RN

Almost all women receiving chemotherapy will experience a change in appetite. Loss of appetite can be made worse when food does not taste the same. Eating habits will frequently be affected. How a person deals with stress will also make an impact on appetite and eating. Make good food choices when you are able to eat because nutrition is important.

Much has been written about diet, health and cancer, and you may now find yourself evaluating your diet. But remember that change doesn't need to happen overnight and may also be difficult at this time. Your desire to make drastic changes in your eating habits, coupled with the advice and urging of others, may only add more stress you certainly don't need. Talk with your physician or nurse if you have a problem with losing or gaining weight. They will evaluate the cause and help you implement steps to correct the problem.

in as usual. I was stunned at the increase in my weight. Of course, I accused the office scales of weighing heavier than my own scales, and the nurse confirmed that other patients had commented on that as well. So I felt comforted that the scale was at fault.

At my next weigh-in, I couldn't believe that I had put on even more weight, although I should have known better. I had been wearing sweatpants throughout the course of treatment for maximum comfort, not to mention the ability to breathe, so I was unaware that I was unable to fit into my real clothes.

I reported this bloated condition to the physician. But after learning of my increased appetite and food consumption, she replied that it was my very own solid tissue that had resulted in weight gain. It was not the result of temporary fluid retention. And I had so hoped for bloat! I wanted the simple way out—a pill to get rid of the bloat and the weight gain without any effort on my part.

I had really become plumper! It took a lot of work to become even a little svelter. I'm still working on it.

I love to eat, my clothes are tight,
Chemo increased my appetite.
I consume three meals then have a snack
And eat chocolate like a maniac.

For those who cannot eat at all
You'll end up looking nice and small.
You'll fit into your clothes with ease
But have a care in a swift breeze.

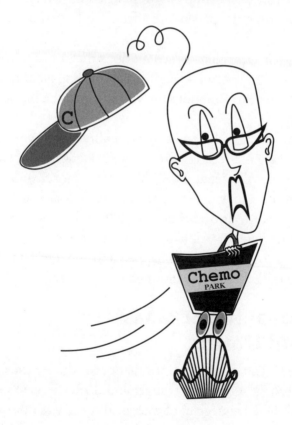

Emotions

3

The period of surgery and the chemotherapy that follows are an emotional time for all who know and love the patient as well as for the patient. It is a time of stress and physical discomfort and a time when some persons share serious thoughts and emotions about life and death.

The patient and her support group all need positive attention and nurturing. Friendship and love make this time more bearable. A phone call, a card, a visit, a dinner delivered, a book, a restaurant lunch, a short scenic car excursion, a ride to chemotherapy are all thoughtful moves that can be made by those who care. Phone calls are almost better than personal visits because they tend to be shorter and don't exhaust the patient.

Cards to family members and friends by other members of the patient's own support group are most welcome. Everyone in the circle surrounding the patient are affected and need positive recognition.

Some days it seems like those emotions that are on a roller coaster trip are hard to control—laughing and feeling good one minute and crying the next. Emotions are very close to the surface and hard to hide.

Some days bring a sharpness to the ability to concentrate. On other days there is a feeling of drifting through life, of being unable to focus on any one detail. I call this occurrence chemo fog. That's not a medical diagnosis, just a personal observation and a symptom that I experienced. It occurs occasionally and randomly. There's just no telling when it will happen. Sometimes I blamed it on exhaustion. Mostly I just let it happen and thought I'd be back to my normal self when the chemotherapy was over.

Emotional Roller Coaster: Ups and Downs

There are a variety of emotions that occur during the course of cancer treatment. Guilt, grief, anger and depression are some of them. And there are degrees of each of those. I was not immune to these up and down feelings.

Some days I felt like I could beat the world. I felt wonderful. I was doing something to save myself. I had my life under control. The discomforts of chemotherapy would be short-lived and would soon pass. I was going for "the cure"!

Some days I could hardly get my chin off my chest. Why did this have to happen to me? I did not deserve this! Those days were tearful. I felt like grieving for myself. What else could I do but have a good cry.

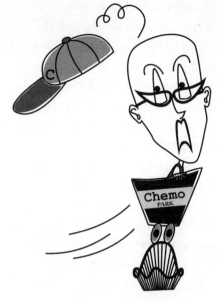

This was worse than PMS—laughing one minute and crying the next.

Some days I didn't feel like being strong. I was the one with the cancer. Why should I be strong for other people? Diverse thoughts went around in my head. One minute I felt like folding up. The next minute I wanted to be strong to make my illness easier on family and friends.

Eventually, I worked at focusing on the positives of the situation. I had access to good medical care. I had a chemotherapy plan that was usually effective. I had a pretty good health record. I was feeling good or at least tolerable. I knew that I could handle this with grace.

So the days went along with my emotions raging up and down. What a difficult period this was! In time, I came to know that I would get through this and come out on the other side stronger and closer to family and friends.

There are degrees of mood swings—from euphoria to severe depression. Some people dwell on having cancer and can't seem to let go of that thought. They become obsessed by it, allowing it to dominate their lives. Although total denial is not a good idea, total absorption is the opposite end of the spectrum.

Guilt is another feeling sometimes experienced. Thoughts like "What did I do to get cancer?" "Is this a punishment for something I did?" That kind of thinking can dominate people's lives. Foremost in their thoughts are their physical symptoms and the discomforts they are experiencing and feel they probably deserve. And they become real Suffering Sallies. These sisters are truly miserable but so are those around them. It rubs off and is difficult to be around.

In these cases and the cases of severe depression, it may be desirable to seek professional counseling to get over the hump. Counseling can be helpful in exploring feelings and getting a hold on them. Many women take antianxiety or antidepression drugs during treatment to help them navigate through this little pothole on the road of life.

There are breast cancer survivor support groups that meet regularly at oncology clinics, community centers or hospitals. Women help each other with feelings and concerns. These groups are led by professional women and are helpful to many participants. In addition, many persons make new and strong friendships with other members of the group. The focus is sharing common experiences and assisting one another to maintain a positive attitude and enjoy each day as much as possible. Information about local groups can be obtained from the nurses at your oncologist's office or from your local library. Also, there are some national resources listed in Appendix B and Appendix D of this book.

The Wig That Almost Escaped

One wintry day, I decided to go to the mall to lift my spirits. I needed the change of scenery. I chose a time when few people would be there. I calculated that to be after the walkers and before the shoppers. I didn't want to be exposed to hordes of people coughing and spreading flu bugs.

I put on my wig and winter coat and off I went. I walked the mall, window-shopped and perused the lovely new items displayed there.

After a time, I headed for my car feeling better with my spirit refreshed. It was a particularly blustery March day, and as I approached my car, the wind whipped up. You guessed it; my wig flew off and blew across the parking lot. There I was Miss Bald Beauty, chasing after it. Lane after lane, it blew until it became wedged under the wheel of a car. I was there in a millisecond, whacking it back into place on my head—gravel, motor oil and all. What a nightmare; exactly what I feared might happen did happen. From this moment on I vowed to wear my new hooded coat. Although I had never worn a hood before, I purchased one specifically for these cold wintry chemotherapy months so I wouldn't catch a cold. At least I figured that wearing my new hooded coat would protect me from a repetition of the flying wig performance.

I was breathless after that run in the parking lot. I held my wig in place as I scrambled into my car. I looked warily around to see if anyone had caught this crazed performance of mine. No one looked back at me. Thank goodness.

As I caught my breath and equilibrium, I thought of how funny I must have looked, scurrying around the parking lot, darting between cars for an object that no one could see. They would have been able to see my bald head, of course, but lots of people seem to be shaving their heads lately—perhaps not middle-aged ladies, but lots of other people.

So maybe it didn't look so strange after all. And what if it did look strange? So what? I would have been the star of someone's dinner joke that evening. That's not so bad. A laugh is a laugh and even I was laughing. I decided to calm down and loosen up. It's only hair and it will come back.

> *Up and down and around I go,*
> *Some days it's really hard to know.*
> *What am I doing on this treatment plan?*
> *And when will my emotions let me land?*
> *I have many feelings and they're all mixed up*
> *But when chemo is over this will all let up.*

Decreased Attention: Chemo Fog

Even on good days, attention span varies from person to person and from chemo to chemo. Some days it may be difficult to concentrate on one task. On other days three tasks can be done at the same time.

I had not heard of chemo fog before I was in the middle of it. When I became distracted and forgetful, I wondered if I was in the midst of developing Alzheimer's disease. Of course, my forgetfulness and a lackadaisical attitude did come on rather suddenly. But I thought if four million Americans suffer from Alzheimer's disease, maybe I'm about to be the four millionth and first!

Once I learned about chemo fog, I began to exploit and enjoy it. It was great! When I'd forget something or lacked interest in something or couldn't figure out something, I just blamed it on chemo fog. It was a great excuse. I used it for as long as I could. Fortunately, this is not a permanent change. I was back to my old self after the treatment cycle was complete. And although I am thankful to be back to normal, now I have no excuse for forgetfulness and inattention.

It should be said that if a person has always been forgetful, disinterested or lack critical thinking skills, these characteristics will not improve after treatment. For better or for worse, chemo recipients return to their former level of function.

I don't remember, I don't know.
Is that important? Do I need to know?
My memory is gone, I can't concentrate.
Thank goodness I'll soon recuperate.

Sleeplessness: The Zombie

In some persons, the steroid medication given before chemotherapy treatments can cause sleeplessness. It acts as a stimulant and transmits a slight feeling of euphoria. Unfortunately, the latter feeling wears off in a few hours.

Worry or anticipation of further illness or unpleasant symptoms may also cause sleeplessness. Sometimes it occurs without explanation. Whatever the cause, the physician can order medication that will aid sleep.

Both sleep and rest are important during the course of chemotherapy. There is a war going on in the body and most of the person's energy is drained by that battle. Rest and sleep replenish that energy. It takes lots of energy to win the war.

So if sleep is elusive, the physician should be informed. With the help of medication, sleeping 10 or 11 hours a night is a real possibility. An afternoon nap might be squeezed in as well. Keep in mind that sleeping after 4 P.M. may increase the difficulty of falling asleep at night. Resting soon after lunch works better if early-to-bed nights are preferred.

Sleeping Beauty

I was one of those who slept only 4 hours each night after my first treatment. This was 4 hours less than I usually slept. I knew that this was not enough to survive gracefully while the chemo war raged on. I felt and moved like a zombie.

I thought I could make sleep happen. The more determined I was, the later sleep came. At bedtime, I tried hot cocoa, hot herbal tea, reading and making lists of what I needed to do in the morning. Nothing worked. Four hours was my maximum sleep even without napping during the daytime. So my oncologist prescribed a mild

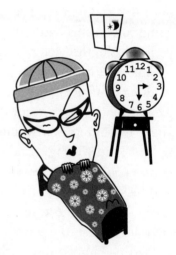

Counting sheep didn't help.

tranquilizer to be taken at bedtime. This was a magic pill! With the help of this mild medication, I slept 8 to 10 hours per night. Loved it! Feeling rested helped me tolerate side effect symptoms with greater grace and composure.

I can't sleep a wink, I don't know why,
I'm all keyed up; I'm ready to cry.
Each day of this treatment is a big test,
But I'm going for the "cure" so I need to rest.
I'll ask the doctor for some "sleepers" to soothe
That will solve this problem and I will rest too.

It's All in the Attitude

A positive attitude makes this whole ghastly situation more tolerable. Maintaining a sense of humor, being able to laugh at yourself and remaining hopeful are pivotal to a successful recovery.

You may not feel like whistling a happy tune every day of the treatment period, but try not to dwell on "How come this happened to me?" and "What did I do to deserve this?" You did nothing to deserve cancer. It was just an accident of nature. Try to block out those thoughts and set your head in the zone that you are going to win this battle. If you find that you cannot do that, tell your oncologist. Many things can be done to help you.

War rages on in every cell of the body while the chemotherapy is working, and all energy is directed to that war. It is more of a struggle for the chemo to work if energy is sapped toward feelings of anger and bitterness. Bucking the fact that the big "C" has reared its ugly head in your body takes a tremendous amount of energy. Of course you may not feel like assuming the role of a cancan dancer and kicking up your lovely heels during the treatment period. But acceptance and the attitude that you will beat this thing are major steps forward in the process of successful treatment.

Getting enough rest during therapy is especially helpful. Some say that chemotherapy works most effectively during sleep. Who knows how that theory developed? But asleep or awake, chemotherapy will work. Your symptoms will verify it.

Another Trip to the Mall

In my attempt to maintain a positive attitude, I made another trip to the mall. I looked forward to another one of these simple outings. I liked the change of scenery and enjoyed seeing what was new and in vogue. In addition, I could walk around a couple of times to get some exercise anonymously. I rarely saw anyone I knew there.

It was a wintry day so I wore my new hooded jacket. I hadn't realized at the time of purchase that the hood was lined with velveteen so it matched the coat. I liked that look. What I didn't think about was that velveteen is a nonslippery fabric. I had purchased the jacket before I lost my hair.

The significance of the nonslippery fabric came to my attention when I put the coat on for the first time while wearing my wig. I attempted to slide the hood forward onto my head but it didn't slide over my wig. Instead the hood pushed the wig along with it so that the wig ended up over my face. At that point I understood that the whole coat had to be lifted in order to position the hood on top of my head and wig. Only with this move could I avoid the sliding-forward action. Alas, there was more to learn.

I got into my car head first and settled myself in the driver's seat. It was a struggle to buckle the seat belt over this quilted coat but finally I was successful.

As I drove along, the permanently mounted headrest continuously pushed the voluminous hood forward, causing the wig to inch forward too until it had moved down to my eyebrows—or at least where my eyebrows used to be. It became uncomfortable and difficult to see as the bangs came precariously close to my eyes. I hoped that no neighboring driver would glance over to see this ridiculously hairy woman manning my mobile. I had no forehead showing, and the wig continued to slip over the previous site of my eyebrows until I was peaking out between the bangs.

I tried to pull off the hood but found it to be an impossible task. The hood was luxuriously large and quilted between its layers of velveteen, and the stationary headrest stood straight up against the hood, moving the wig continuously forward. I was trapped and near tears. It was a constant wrestling match with the wig and the hood and the permanently affixed headrest as I tried to maneuver them while struggling to maintain control of the car.

I made it to the parking lot and removed the hood as soon as I alighted from my car. After a while, I became less agitated from my adventurous ride and my mood began to lighten up. When I was ready to leave, for some unknown reason, I entered my car right hip first. I usually stick my head in the car first but this was a different day in many ways. Wow! I cracked my head so hard on the door frame that I thought I might have a concussion. I saw stars! And my sore head was hanging out of the car! There was not enough room to move my head into the car with the wig and the gigantic padded hood. I had to get out of the car, turn around and get in head first. It was quite a struggle. From then on, I moved the seat back after parking to facilitate the exit and entry processes.

It was difficult for me to maintain a positive attitude with a possible concussion, a headache and a wig in my eyes. On some days, nothing is easy. Life seems like such a struggle!

At the time, this whole scenario wasn't funny to me. But looking back at the whole incident, it struck me that this would have been a great silent movie. A film showing myself struggling to get in and out of a car, cracking my head, and peeking through my wig as the hood slipped over my forehead, would have brought the house down with laughter in the 1920s.

Fears

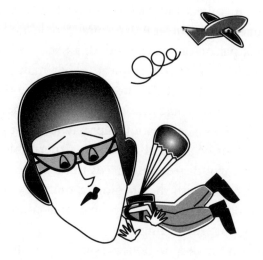

o many fears go through the mind of a person who has experienced cancer and chemotherapy. Much is related to age, sex, the location and extent of the cancer, and situation in life—such as if the person is in a relationship, if the person is a stay-at-home mom or if the person is the main breadwinner.

Some patients can talk about their fears to family members, friends, medical persons or to a cancer support group. Some persons choose not to talk of them at all. But some fears are usually present.

My initial fears included several facets. What was the extent of the cancer? Had it metastasized? Would it recur? Would I live to see a grandchild? How long would I be able to care for myself? Where would I go to live if I became too weak to live alone in my home? Would I become a burden to my children?

Both my family members and friends gathered around and were very supportive of me. But I realize that some people are uncomfortable with a sick person or, heaven forbid, a person who is dying. Those persons cannot visit or communicate. They may see themselves in that afflicted friend, or the situation may remind them of their own mortality. So they just cannot tolerate being near.

A person who is in a sexual relationship may feel that the change in appearance may not be acceptable to the partner. This may precipitate much emotional distress and needs to be addressed. Discussing these feelings with the oncologist, oncology nurse, cancer support group or seeking ongoing professional counseling may be helpful to bring out true feelings.

My niece's husband makes no bones about his love for his wife. He tells her repeatedly that it is she whom he loves and he wants her to be well. The appearance of the mastectomy scar and her choice of not having reconstruction do not bother him. He loves her for herself. That must be very comforting for my niece to hear.

Sometimes, friends and family members offer to help. Let them. Of course, if you were the person who did the chores around the house before the chemo, your husband, partner or children or friends may not be aware of what needs to be done without some guidance from you. For instance, someone else may not notice that the kitchen floor needs to be washed until their shoes stick to it. And even then, if they walk fast, only your shoes will be sticking to the floor. So make a list.

Setting a Goal

A patient of mine who was seriously ill with untreatable ovarian cancer wanted to live to see her daughter married. Much to the amazement of the medical community, she beat the odds and lived to attend the wedding. She set her mind and it saved her until the wedding. She attended the wedding in grand style then died shortly thereafter. The power of the mind is astounding.

One of my favorite patients was a 5-year-old boy who had his leg amputated because of bone cancer. One day, I found him crying in his bed. Naturally, I thought he was crying because his leg was gone. But he told me that he wasn't worried about that because he knew that he would get a wooden leg. His fears concerned wearing his wooden leg to swim and if that leg would float. It turned out that before his surgery, his older brother had been teaching him to swim and he didn't want to give up that important connection with this brother, whom he idolized.

Lisa Silipo, a lovely young woman in her late 20s, was diagnosed with breast cancer just as she was getting ready to finish her masters degree in education. She had spent years working hard in school and was excited to begin an internship working with high school students. "Never in a million years" could she have believed that she would be diagnosed with stage II breast cancer before the end of her last semester. Graduation was scheduled for mid-May, and on April 6th she received the diagnosis. Although the news was a major setback, Lisa decided she had worked hard to get where she was and was determined to graduate "come hell or high water!" She knew that it would be too easy to let fear make her a recluse, and somewhere deep in her soul she knew she could not let this happen. She continued with her internship, supported by her husband, family and friends. Graduation gave her a reason to keep on going and to "beat this horrible disease." Finally, in May, with all of her family watching, she walked across the stage and received her diploma. Of all of the hundreds of people in attendance that day, only a few knew that Lisa was in the beginning stages of the biggest battle of her life! Looking back now, Lisa believes that completing her education allowed her to look ahead and see that she still had a future.

It helps to allow patients to bring up their own concerns because they may be on topics that you'd never have guessed, and sharing them may be a source of great relief to the individual.

Making Fear Manageable

By Barbara Tripp, RN

The feeling of fear is universal. We all have fears. The feeling ranges from a subtle sense of uneasiness to absolute panic. Some of us share our fears easily and others have learned to hide the feeling behind a masterfully created facade. At times, we are able to control our fears, while at other times, perhaps when we least expect it, the fear controls us. This is especially true when dealing with a diagnosis of cancer. The greatest fear for most people in this situation is fear of the unknown. Sometimes it is hard to articulate exactly what we are afraid of. Separating the fear into components that are perhaps more manageable may be helpful. One woman who was a patient of mine would repeat over and over "I'm so scared, I'm so scared." It took time for her to list the things she was afraid of. Once we had a list to work from, we could tackle one item at a time and actually eliminate some of her fears and develop strategies to deal with others.

The fear of death and leaving loved ones is on almost everyone's list. I have found in my practice that once this fear has been put into words and said out loud, patients feel a sense of freedom, a sense of being in control, or at least regaining some control, over their emotions.

Many women cancer patients also feel like they have lost control of their lives. Something else is in charge. Regaining a sense of control of their lives is hard work, and acknowledging what they don't have control over is also key in this process. It is good to remember that absolute control over anything is an illusion.

Another Decision

One of the young women I know has a grim family history of breast cancer. In fact, none of the women in her family survived to see their oldest child live beyond their fourth year. They all died of breast cancer. With that family history, she feared that the same would happen to her. She had young children and she wanted to live to see them grow to adult-

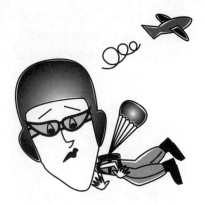

I tried not to let fears of what I couldn't control get me down.

hood. And she wanted to live to become a grandmother.

So she, her husband and her physician conferred together and decided that the safest course of action was for her to have prophylactic mastectomies. This action would prevent breast cancer from developing. She selected reconstructive surgery as well.

Her husband said that he loves her so much that he wants her healthy and in his life. He was very supportive throughout the ordeal and has been her mainstay. She did not need chemotherapy, however, because she did not have cancer.

Body Image

The appearance of one's body is very important to some women. Many of us look at the latest magazines and wish that we had the body of one of the models or movie stars pictured there. We may even fantasize about how our lives might be different if we had a beautiful body. Also, there is the concern that a husband or partner will no longer find the woman attractive after surgery.

A surgery that changes the appearance of a person may be viewed as a catastrophe. Some women have even refused surgery to remove the breast cancer because they did not want to accept the disfigurement it causes. People don't seem to mind having surgery that doesn't change the body's external appearance, such as having a gallbladder or appendix removed. But when appearance is involved, they may hesitate. Refusing a mastectomy to remove a cancer is unwise because the cancer will continue to grow and eventually take the life of the person.

We all want to feel good about ourselves and the way we look. It is especially important to look good to our mate or significant other.

Reconstructive Surgery

By Barbara Tripp, RN

Although lumpectomy followed by radiation is a safe and effective option for some women, a mastectomy may be the recommended surgical treatment. Any procedure that results in a change in the woman's appearance will require physical and psychological adjustment. A person's self-esteem can be affected by outward appearance, and a woman's sense of identity as it relates to femininity and sexuality is part of her body image. To minimize the physical changes caused by the mastectomy, some women choose reconstructive surgery. Before choosing reconstructive surgery, however, it is important to discuss all of the available options and their associated risks and benefits with a plastic surgeon.

Finding a plastic surgeon who specializes in breast reconstruction following mastectomy is also important. This may take some time and perhaps include some travel, but it will be worth your time and effort. Many breast surgeons work closely with plastic surgeons and can be one resource for the referral. You should also consider having a consultation with a plastic surgeon before the mastectomy because that feedback may help you make a decision regarding reconstruction, increase your reconstructive options postoperatively and provide psychological comfort during this already-stressful time.

There is no right or wrong decision when considering reconstruction. Your goal should be to make the best decision for yourself. Gathering information, consulting health care professionals with specialized knowledge in reconstruction, talking with a husband or partner and speaking with other women who have also had to make this decision are some strategies that will assist you in making the decision. There are so many things to think about and do when you first learn about your diagnosis. Some women leave the discussion about reconstruction for after treatment, believing the life and death issues need to happen first. However, one more appointment may also help your peace of mind now and increase your options later.

I have a dear friend who did well after her mastectomy and throughout her chemotherapy treatments. Her husband also seemed very supportive. When at last her hair began to grow, she was ecstatic.

One Sunday, as she prepared to go to church with her husband, she showered, shampooed, moussed and blow dried her 2-inch-long hair. She was so proud of it and felt so good when she came out of the bathroom. She said to her husband, "I think I won't wear my wig today." He was quiet for a moment as he looked at her and then he said, "I think you should wear your wig."

The day after she told me her story, I sent a mood ring to her along with a warning for my friend to tell her husband. It goes like this: "I received a mood ring from my friend today. She said to tell you that when I'm in a good mood it will turn green. When I'm in a bad mood because of something you've said to me, it will leave a red mark on your forehead." Hm! I guess not everyone is capable of moral support. Some days it seems as though we need to keep our own morale up.

Reoccurrence: Metastasis

Because of the nature and ability of the cancer to recur or travel to other organs, reoccurrence is a natural concern. Following the treatment plan and following up with the required examinations and tests are the best plan to prevent this from occurring.

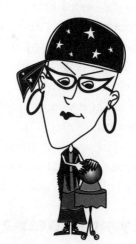

Some kinds of cancer cells are more prone to recur and travel. This needs to be discussed with the oncologist, and the most appropriate health plan needs to be determined.

Future Risks

None of us knows what the future holds. As I see it, anyone can keel over at any moment. Fortunately, most of us

Nightly attempts to predict the future only deprived me of beauty sleep.

What Is Metastasis?

By Joanna Brell, MD

Metastasis refers to the spread of a cancer outside the body part it originated from and beyond the lymph nodes surrounding that body part. Breast cancer is considered to have metastasized if it is found in any solid organ such as the liver, lungs, bone or brain. Metastatic breast cancer is often fatal. Based on certain characteristics of the tumor, it is possible to estimate the risk of developing metastatic disease. Most women can have their risk reduced by taking chemotherapy, hormonal therapy or both. Although at this time, there are no other ways to decrease the risk of developing metastases, these medications can kill any microscopic tumor cells that may still be in the bloodstream after surgery. Radiation therapy and surgery are unable to attack these circulating cells because they have no effect on the bloodstream. Women must discuss their individual risk with their doctor, as there are many factors that determine the level of risk.

don't. I've decided that worrying about something that is not in my control is wasting my energy and spoiling the day I am living.

I try to follow reasonable guidelines for healthy living and hope for the best. I know I could be doing more, like increasing the amount of exercise I do each day, but I don't lie awake worrying about it. I need my beauty sleep.

I have two daughters who are worried about developing breast cancer. I was the first person in my family to have breast cancer so I look at it as a random happening. But I warn them to take precautions.

They are both mid-30s. They do breast self-exams, have an annual physical exam and mammograms as prescribed. But they are still fearful about developing breast cancer.

Lymphedema

Lymphedema is a concern if most of the lymph nodes have been removed from the underarm. Because the lymphatic fluid seeks to

Is Breast Cancer Hereditary?

By Joanna Brell, MD

Only 10 percent of breast cancer is considered hereditary, and there are several genes that have been implicated in passing this risk of cancer among family members. Of current interest, the BRCA1 or 2 genes impart a 50 to 85 percent lifetime risk of developing breast carcinoma. Because of this risk, a woman or man should know if they are carriers of these genes, especially because there are interventions, such as prophylactic surgery or medications, that can substantially reduce this risk.

Who is at risk to inherit these genes? Hereditary breast cancer has some very characteristic features. It almost always occurs at an early (premenopausal) age and often strikes both breasts. First-degree relatives (mother, daughters, sisters) will also have breast cancer. If one has a postmenopausal first-degree relative with breast cancer or is the first in the family to be afflicted, it is unlikely to be hereditary cancer. A first-degree relative does increase one's risk of developing breast cancer by a few percent.

Unfortunately, the majority of breast cancers are considered sporadic or without identifiable cause and are unrelated to these genes. It is prohibitive to test and counsel everyone for these genes; there are numerous other genes and factors related to the development of breast carcinoma that are yet unknown, so universal testing may give a false sense of security.

Your oncologist can decide if there is a genetic link. If there is, a family member with breast cancer must first have the blood test; if the blood test turns out to be positive, then other members may be tested and counseled. If it is negative, no further testing is needed at this time.

return from the cells in the arm and there are no nodes under the arm to carry it away, the arm on the mastectomy side of the body may become swollen.

If lymphedema occurs, there are special exercises that can be recommended by a physical therapist to minimize or prevent this problem from worsening. In addition, there is an elastic glove and

> **LYMPH:** The liquid portion of the blood that comes out of the small blood vessels to bathe and nourish each cell.
> **EDEMA:** Retention of fluid or swelling.

an arm cuff that can be worn periodically. The arm cuff is much like a blood pressure cuff that inflates and deflates to encourage the edema to pass out of the arm.

Lymphedema

By Joanna Brell, MD

The risk of lymphedema after axillary lymph node dissection is much less than 10 percent for most women. Many health care centers offer educational and treatment programs on lymphedema management through the occupational therapy department. In general, recommendations for preventing arm swelling include returning to full exercise after surgery; this should occur gradually with instruction from the surgeon and lymphedema specialist. The skin of the affected arm should be kept clean and moist to decrease the risk of infection resulting from dry skin. One must monitor the arm and hand for infection and swelling, seeking guidance early if these conditions develop.

Nerve Damage

There are many structures under the arm besides the lymph nodes. Muscles and nerves are two of them. Sometimes lymph nodes are curled around a nerve that might be severed or damaged during the surgery. This is an unusual occurrence but it has happened. In this case, physical therapy may be part of the recovery plan. The physician and patient will determine the best treatment for the condition.

5

Digestive Ups and Downs

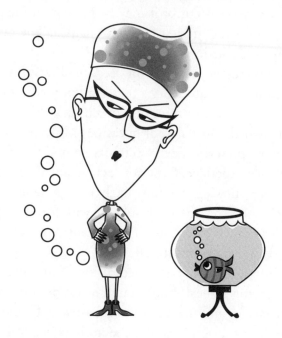

Chemotherapy wreaks havoc on many body systems, but perhaps the most difficult to deal with is the digestive system. For a person who loves to eat, this can be especially distressing. Nausea, vomiting, diarrhea, constipation and flatus are the most distressing gastrointestinal symptoms.

Nausea and Vomiting: Queasiness and Upchucking

Initially, to prevent the occurrence of nausea, I was given antinausea medication intravenously before the administration of chemotherapy.

In the weeks following each administration of the chemo drugs, nausea may occur in a variety of frequencies and intensities. However, it may never occur or it may be present all the time. On a scale, queasiness is the mildest feeling of nausea. The maximum feeling of nausea results in vomiting.

Nausea may be slight and occur in occasional waves or it may be severe and constant. An antinausea prescription medication such as Compazine can be taken to minimize or alleviate this symptom. It should be taken at the first sign of queasiness. In cases of severe nausea, it may be prescribed every 6 hours around the clock. Persons who have experienced motion sickness or who were nauseated during pregnancy are the most likely to experience nausea during the course of treatment. It may be wise for these persons to take the medication every 6 hours as a preventive measure, at least during the first week after treatment.

As stated, if nausea occurs, the medication should be taken immediately. Trying to beat it and tough it out doesn't usually work. Misery ensues and maybe vomiting as well. The medication does not interrupt the action of the chemotherapy and it is recommended by oncologists.

Antinausea medication is usually taken by mouth, but if nausea is severe and vomiting is a possibility or a fact, suppositories may be prescribed.

Coping with Nausea

Some days I was unsure of the presence of nausea. It was not an overt kind of symptom. I moved carefully so as not to precipitate it. Also, I wasn't certain how my gastrointestinal tract would behave after each chemo so I postponed any social plans.

Sometimes, occasional waves of nausea or worse determined my day. On those days, I stayed at home just having a "bathroom kind of day" until I felt more sure of my status and the "almost feeling" of queasiness passed.

I feel like I'm on a rolling ship
My tummy is asking, "Why this trip?"
I must get off this boat or I will see
My favorite cookies and my latest tea.
I will take a pill to help with this queaze
Then consume more calories with greater ease.

Vomiting

Vomiting was my least favorite activity although I usually felt better after it happened. It just wasn't any fun. I worked at trying to be thankful for commodes and indoor plumbing. Life must not have been easy during the era of the outhouse although that was before my time. During each upchuck, I reminded myself that things could have been worse.

Some people never vomit after chemotherapy. Some vomit every day. Some vomit only during the middle week of each 3-week cycle when they were most vulnerable. Some vomit the day chemo is administered and up to 72 hours after, then not again until after the next chemo.

An antiemetic drug can be helpful to prevent vomiting. A pillow to kneel on and a soft toilet seat make the experience more tolerable. But it is never easy or pleasant.

If vomiting is a possibility, consuming small meals more than three times a day can be helpful. Also, not eating or drinking anything during the period of nausea and immediately after vomiting

Why Chemotherapy May Cause Vomiting

By Joanna Brell, MD

Chemotherapy causes vomiting because of several mechanisms. It can destroy the lining of the stomach and entire gastrointestinal tract so that digestion is more difficult and acid production is higher. In addition, the chemo and its by-products circulate in the blood and stimulate the areas of the brain that control the process of vomiting. Also, the anxiety that people feel from their diagnosis and subsequent treatment can produce nausea. Sometimes the cancer itself can make proteins that induce nausea and vomiting.

helps to minimize more upchucking. When the stomach and intestine are moving in reverse, eating and drinking only stimulate more vomiting.

Antinausea medication needs to stay down if it is going to be helpful. Swallowing the pill with only a tiny bit of water serves to sneak up on the stomach. Hopefully, it will not be aware that something new has been introduced and vomit it back up.

Rinsing the mouth with water and brushing the teeth are usually enough to freshen the mouth. Strong commercial mouthwashes should be avoided. They are too harsh and can encourage mouth sores to develop.

Now I know what life in the fast lane is. It's a chemo survivor dashing to the bathroom to hang over the commode. Sometimes this vomiting symptom "comes up" so quickly, almost without warning. There is no time for discussion or explanations, only time to get to the facilities to avoid an unexpected and embarrassing accident.

It is important to consume fluids even during bouts of nausea and vomiting. Small sips of water, tea or bouillon may stay down. Dehydration and electrolyte imbalances should be avoided. If constant vomiting is occurring, the oncologist should be notified. Occasionally, intravenous fluids may be needed but usually the antinausea medication can be changed or the dose increased until the vomiting is under control.

Solving the Dash-to-the-Bath Problem

Some days, I found that it was not advisable to leave the bathroom area. On those days, I'd just place a magazine or book in there and remain in the vicinity. It seemed like too much effort to leave the area then have the need to speed back for the big event. I found it safer to be nearby.

A common view at my abode
Is inside the bowl of my commode.
It has become a familiar sight
Because this chemo is such a fight.
But if I should lose my lunch today
Nausea pills will make my dinner stay.
I'll not let this upchucking get me down
I'm thinking "cure" and out on the town.

Tips on Foods	
To Minimize Nausea and Vomiting	**May Cause Nausea and Vomiting**
Eat cool bland foods, such as eggs, pasta with butter and cheese, Cream of Wheat, cereal, custard, Jell-O, potatoes, pears, bananas	Foods with strong odors, such as garlic, onions, fish
Take small, frequent feedings	Eating three large meals per day
Take nourishing liquids 60 minutes before meals	Minimizing liquids at meals to save room for solid food
Take antinausea medication 30 minutes before meal	Not taking the antinausea medication
Use few spices in foods	Eating highly spiced foods

Diarrhea: The Runs

Diarrhea may or may not occur after chemotherapy. Instead, stools may be soft and passed frequently during the day. Your physician will probably want to be notified if you pass more than three stools per day.

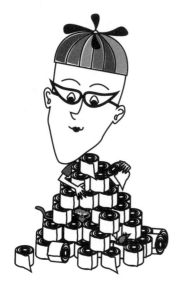

If diarrhea does occur, avoid foods that have precipitated this symptom in the past. Chemo doesn't change past habits. If gravy or chocolate caused diarrhea before chemo, it will cause it during and after chemo as well. If soft, frequent or liquid stools occur, avoid foods that increase activity of the intestine such as roughage and foods containing bran.

If diarrhea occurs, the physician should be notified. Medications are available to minimize or eliminate this symptom. Prolonged diarrhea can alter the normal balance of sodium, potassium and other elements in the system. This can result in serious medical conditions.

Stock up on supplies. Who says diamonds are a girl's best friend?

Placing a calendar in the bathroom facilitates keeping track of defecations and other symptoms as they develop. When it's time to meet with the oncologist, a summary of happenings can be made using this calendar as a guide.

A Hazardous Position

I learned to my dismay that my idea of comfort in bed could be hazardous to my health. I was particularly conscious of positioning the overinflated tissue expander on the mastectomy side because it was hard and uncomfortable to lie on.

To add to my comfort, I share my bed with a body pillow. I use it to prop my arm and leg when lying on my side—my favorite position. After positioning the contour pillow for my head, a foam pillow for my torso (below my remaining breast and the expander) and the body pillow along the side of the mattress, there is barely enough room for myself.

But each night I would climb in and tuck the sheet, electric blanket and quilt around me—no easy feat as I lay on my side. But it was worth it once I got situated. The hazardous part came when nature made an emergency bathroom call. I almost broke my neck getting untangled and out of bed before the runs occurred! I felt like Harry Houdini getting out of his elaborate encasements with great speed but with much less flair and without a drum roll.

> *I can't trust myself to leave my home*
> *I'll have to communicate by phone.*
> *The frequency of nature's call*
> *Prevents my visiting the mall.*
> *I don't feel like going anywhere*
> *Except to bed in my own sweet lair.*

Gas: The Flatus Factory

Accompanying the increase in the rate of defecation and the possible occurrence of diarrhea comes an increase in flatus and associated gas pains. These pains can be severe—so severe, in fact, that they can be mistaken for a heart attack. They move around, travel across the abdomen and downward toward the exit. They can radi-

Why Chemotherapy May Cause Constipation

By Joanna Brell, MD

Some, but not all, chemotherapies can directly affect the small nerves of the gastrointestinal tract. These nerves maintain the normal motion of the gut, so that food and waste may pass through the system appropriately. If these nerves are slowed by treatment, constipation will occur; occasionally, this can also cause nausea and vomiting. People need to use combinations of stool softeners and laxatives (usually every day), drink lots of water and exercise to have a bowel movement every 2 to 3 days.

ate to the shoulder blades. They can be sharp and unrelenting. They can take your breath away.

The different characteristics between gas pains and heart pains help determine the source of the pain and the next step; that is, to wait until the flatus passes or to call 911. Heart problems cause a pressure, tightness or pain in the middle of the chest, sometimes radiating into the jaw, left shoulder or left arm. The pain lasts more than 2 minutes. A heart attack causes a rapid pulse and a cold sweat, except that sweat glands don't function during chemotherapy. Flatus results in a roving pain. Both can be sharp and severe.

The abdominal pain most experienced during the course of chemotherapy is caused by gas, so patience and tolerance are key. Gas pains don't last long. They usually pass in a few minutes and they don't occur frequently. However, some days you may feel like a flatus factory, seemingly to have no end to it.

There are commercial products on the market to minimize the production of flatus. Beano and Gas-X are two of them and I have been told that they are effective. Armed with those medications, venturing out will be less worrisome because there might be more than gas expelled during ejection of flatus.

Some say that a warm water bottle or heating pad set to low heat and applied to the abdomen may help. At least it will make you feel like you are doing something for yourself.

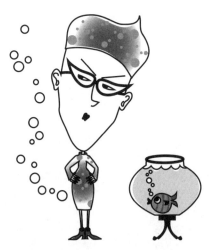

Hopefully this problem didn't affect the ozone.

I have also been told that the consumption of a peppermint LifeSaver (with real sugar, not sugarless) may be used as a differentiating test. Gas will dissipate after sucking this lozenge and the pains will disappear, whereas heart pains will not.

However, if there is any question about having heart attack, calling 911 is the safest course of action. The paramedics will understand if you expel a little flatus en route to the emergency room.

An Untimely Excursion

During the course of my chemotherapy, I needed to make a brief trip to the bank. I timed this carefully between bathroom visits and wore a long coat in the event of a flatus expulsion. I didn't want to draw attention to such a sensory event.

When I arrived at the bank, there appeared to be hordes of people already waiting in line. My mistake. I hadn't considered the date. I didn't remember that during the first few days of the month, some of those persons who receive Social Security checks by mail deposit them in person.

I got in line but it didn't move. I looked at the tellers' windows and noticed that there was only one teller working. I couldn't believe my eyes! I began working up a head of steam about the unfairness of the situation. Certainly, every bank manager knows that this Social Security phenomenon happens at the beginning of every month. More tellers should have been scheduled to work!

Then I thought that perhaps there might be several tellers working but they'd all gone on breaks together. I was enraged! How could a service industry serve the public in such a thoughtless manner? This was infuriating!

Shortly after I had worked myself into a near apoplectic state, I noticed a young man walking out of the bank with a paper bag under his arm. He was the only person who had been waited on the whole time I was there. As soon as he was out the door, it automatically locked and four tellers' heads appeared from under the counter! It turned out that the young man who had just left had robbed the bank! When he requested funds from the teller, she buzzed a silent signal to her fellow tellers and the security videotape began to roll. At the silent alarm, the tellers disappeared under the bulletproof counter. I almost had more than flatus at discovering the real story! My quick trip to the bank turned out to be more of an adventure than I'd ever wanted or anticipated. I hope they recorded my good side on that videotape. Maybe viewing my breath-taking beauty will distract them from my angry face.

Such sound effects and odorous noise
Would disrupt any woman's social poise.
I'm bent over in pain as the gas goes by
I sometimes even want to cry.
I hope that this symptom too will pass
I've never had this volume of gas.

Double Urination: Pee Pee

Some women experience double urination in one "sitting." That is, after voiding they feel that their bladder is empty and they are finished. Then they are surprised because a strong urge to urinate returns almost immediately, sometimes before they leave the bathroom, sometimes after. This is called double urination or pee pee because the bladder doesn't completely empty at the first void and the residual urine is right there ready to flow. So two voidings happen at one sitting.

Those who experience this symptom will want to stay close to the bathroom or remain seated until the second stream of urine is complete. When away from home, it might be wise to wear a pantiliner to catch any drips from slight incontinence after urination.

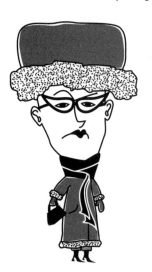

If pantiliners are worn daily or frequently, using a breathable pad allows air circulation and helps prevent the development of a vaginal discharge. I found that Poise and Serenity pads worked best for me. They held the urine without soaking through and without odor.

This double urination can last for a few days or throughout the course of treatment. Fortunately, this is not a permanent change. It ends when chemotherapy is complete.

Pink Urine

I was slowed down by mental telepathy between my bladder and coat.

Another interesting facet to add to the routine procedure of voiding is the color

Why Chemotherapy May Cause Changes in Urination

By Joanna Brell, MD

Deviations from the normal patterns of urination are common when undergoing chemotherapy for a variety of reasons. Bladder infections happen more frequently. Often, people will eat and drink more or less than usual, causing more or less urine production. Some medications can irritate the lining of the bladder and cause inflammation and bleeding. It is also likely that minor irritation occurs, causing some low-grade muscle spasms and the need to eliminate urine more often. The mind and the bladder are intimately linked and it is easy to maintain these nonharmful urinary changes.

of urine. This can also become another source of worry if you are uninformed.

The chemotherapy agent Adriamycin is pink in color. It is excreted through the kidneys. Thus, following its administration, your urine will be pink in color for a few hours. Again, this is not a permanent change.

Doing Double Duty

During the course of chemotherapy, I learned that I had a very unusual bladder. It had mental telepathy with my coat. I know this because as soon as I'd don my coat, scarf, hat and gloves, I'd have to return to the bathroom. It was the most amazing phenomenon. This scenario began after my first chemo treatment so I blamed it on those toxic chemicals.

This was not a disastrous symptom, but it did slow me down and continued to do so over a period of time. I learned that all symptoms disappear eventually but some take longer than others to do so. In my case, I could hardly wait for this pee pee side effect to pass! I hoped for quicker exits.

The strangest thing has happened to me
When I think that I have finished with pee.

It comes again and quite a bit
I should learn to relax and sit.
I'll keep a book close by to read
Until the residual is peed.

Physiological Changes

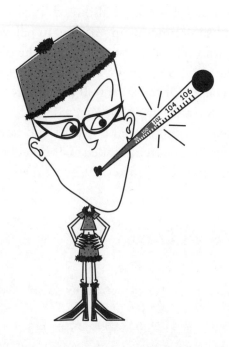

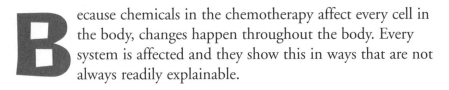

Because chemicals in the chemotherapy affect every cell in the body, changes happen throughout the body. Every system is affected and they show this in ways that are not always readily explainable.

Dry Mouth: Cottonmouth

Some women experience dry mouth during chemotherapy. It feels like there is cotton in the mouth soaking up all the saliva. I was one of those women. It began during the second week after receiving the first treatment and occurred periodically after that. I knew that all glandular activity was suppressed by chemo, so I shouldn't have been surprised that the salivary glands were depressed as well. The result of this lack of saliva production was less liquid in my mouth.

I tried drinking lots of fluid and sucking on lots of ice cubes to relieve that cottonmouth feeling. I also used lip gloss, a petroleum-based lipstick and sometimes plain Vaseline to relieve my dry lips.

Another symptom that often occurs during the course of treatment is a metallic taste. Some days, everything that went into my mouth tasted metallic. Of those 10,000 taste buds I harbored, I thought that 9,998 must have been affected.

I discovered that sucking frozen popsicles and flavored ice cubes temporarily relieved this taste. I made small ice cubes with Kool-Aid and lemonade powdered mixes. When I made these cubes, I

Why Taste Buds Change

By Joanna Brell, MD

Usually, it is medications that change taste. Chemo kills fast-growing cells such as cancer and hair and taste buds. The taste buds may be temporarily stunned and people experience aversions and new preferences. Heightened sensitivity to bitter tastes commonly occurs; therefore, many people avoid coffee, meats, chocolate and tomatoes. The mind influences taste very much, and some people never regain their taste for pretreatment favorites.

used only half of the suggested liquid recommended in the recipe. Thus the flavor was more concentrated and the metallic taste was better relieved. I used trays with semicircular-shaped cups to provide contoured cubes that were more comfortable in my mouth. I found that orange-flavored Kool-Aid cubes were especially effective in relieving the metallic taste, and lemonade cubes were particularly refreshing.

Another trick that helped relieve that metallic taste was sucking soft, flavorful candies, such as Gummi Savers, made by Lifesavers. I ate bags of them—not many calories but lots of flavor.

Silent Days

I have never been as quiet as I was during my chemotherapy. My mouth was so dry! I had no saliva. I found it extremely difficult to talk with my tongue stuck to the roof of my mouth. Some days, I felt like I had to pry it loose with my fingers.

I found that increasing my fluid intake helped a little. But even after the course of chemotherapy was complete, all glandular secretion continued to be suppressed for several months. There was not much to be done that was really effective. At least I could be thankful that I had no ring-around-the-collar because my oil glands were suppressed as well.

> *I remember when I used to be*
> *A woman who talked incessantly.*
> *But since my mouth is now so dry*
> *I can't even sing a lullaby.*
> *Though I've learned a lot by hearing others*
> *I'd talk a lot if I had my druthers.*

Sore Mouth: Mucositis

During the second or third week after treatment, many people experience open sores in their mouths or throats, or find that the lining of their mouths and throats has reddened. These sores may be external or internal. External sores can be seen. They are located on the inside of the cheek or under the tongue. Internal sores

> **MUCOSITIS:** The medical name for swelling of a mucous membrane.
> **ASPIRATION:** To inhale food or fluid—sometimes referred to as "down the wrong pipe."

resemble blood blisters and occur inside the tongue. Internal sores are not usually visible but their pain is certainly felt. In may be necessary to eat soft foods with little or no spices. Warm soup and ice cream are comforting. Rough foods and hot temperatures increase the irritation.

Open sores can be treated with a prescription mouthwash that numbs the inside of the mouth and an over-the-counter antiseptic throat spray that numbs the throat. Be sure to ask the physician for something to alleviate this symptom.

While the mouth or throat is numb, care must be taken when swallowing to avoid aspiration. The numbness produced by these solutions is only temporary and the relief lasts only a short time. Mouth and throat sores usually heal before it is time for the next chemo treatment.

A Closer Look at Mucositis

By Joanna Brell, MD

Mucous membranes line the mouth and the entire gastrointestinal tract as well as the respiratory and genitourinary systems. Because the mucous membranes have a short life span and are composed of fast-growing cells, chemotherapy can easily inhibit their constant renewal process.

Mucositis occurs predictably with many chemotherapy treatments and is the result of loss of the membranes as well as inflammation. Sores develop because the mucous membranes are now unable to protect the mouth from bacteria and other invaders. The inflammation causes pain, the mouth is dry and there may be bleeding. Meticulous mouth care can very much diminish these problems and pain medicines used only in the mouth and those that are swallowed are effective. If mucositis develops, preventative care should start the day of the next chemotherapy cycle.

Tooth Decay: Crowned Again

One of the lesser-known side effects of chemotherapy is tooth decay. The good news is that it can be prevented.

Tooth decay occurs because of the decrease in saliva production. Because the mouth is so dry, food particles stick to the teeth and are not washed away by saliva as is usually the case.

There are special prescription dental creams available on the market to prevent this decay from happening. One of them is PreviDent 5000 Plus. It contains a higher concentration of fluoride than the over-the-counter creams available commercially.

This prescription toothpaste should be used at bedtime. It works all night. It should be applied after brushing with regular toothpaste and after thorough rinsing. Eating and drinking after applying the special paste will rub it off, rendering it ineffective.

A Detour to the Dentist

I was scheduled for a mastectomy on a Thursday morning. The previous Monday, I awoke with a massive toothache. Oh, boy! Did

XEROSTOMIA: Means dry mouth from decreased saliva..

How Is Chemotherapy Related to Tooth Decay?

By Joanna Brell, MD

Mucositis also accelerates tooth decay, as will any process that decreases saliva production. It increases oral bacteria and causes mouth pain so that usual dental care is too painful to perform. Dry mouth from decreased saliva is called xerostomia and occurs when chemotherapy and other medications prevent the salivary glands from functioning proficiently. Keeping the mouth moist and stimulating the salivary glands are the most helpful measures in preventing mucositis and, therefore, tooth decay. You will need to avoid anything that irritates the mouth, including alcohol, which is found in most mouthwashes.

it hurt! I thought that this must be some kind of test or distraction to divert my attention from the main event. It was just too ludicrous to be happening.

Off I went to my dentist for an emergency visit. Oh, yes. A root canal was needed for an infection in the tooth's root system and my jawbone. To go into surgery with an infection already in progress was not my notion of ideal. And yet I didn't want to postpone the surgery because I didn't want the cancer to get me. What a dilemma.

So I began the course of antibiotics on Monday, had the root canal on Tuesday, had a temporary crown put in place on Wednesday and the mastectomy on Thursday. I can think of better ways to spend a week.

At least the dental cream worked for me. I still have all of my own teeth with their root canals and crowns. And during that important week in my life, I was crowned again. Maybe there's a message there.

> *I've always loved my pearly whites*
> *I whiten them to keep them bright.*
> *They even twinkle in the night*
> *Plus they enable me to chew and bite.*
>
> *Every day I floss and fluorinate*
> *'Cause my teeth help me to articulate.*
> *They're all my own both up and down*
> *Including that root canal and crown.*

Vision Changes: Bleary Eyed

Vision changes can occur anytime during the course of chemotherapy. Most of them last only a few hours to a day and occur periodically without warning.

At times my eyes felt hot and dry. I learned that this was not harmful to the eyes but it certainly was uncomfortable. Although it lasted only a few hours, it came and went during the course of treatment. I used artificial tears to moisten my eyes and facilitate blinking—and winking.

Another symptom that I found troubling was my eyes pooling with tears. That resulted in the sensation that I was looking through water. Because this symptom caused blurred and bleary vision, I turned to large-print library books to prevent eyestrain.

Sometimes the tears spilled over and ran down my face. During the night, tears pooled at the inner corners of my eyes, creating big puddles by morning. I was surprised at this because most of the rest of my glands had dried up and stopped secreting.

Occasionally I was visited by the sand-man. I would awaken to find myself rub-bing the sand from my lids. That sand was a result of dead cells gathering at the base of my lashes. On arising, I used diluted baby shampoo on my index fingers to rub away those dead cells, then rinsed with a wash-cloth and warm water.

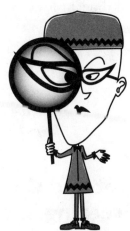

Sometimes I couldn't even find my glasses.

Of all the symptoms that I experienced pertaining to my eyes, I found cloudy vision to be the most troubling. I felt like I had suddenly developed advanced cataracts or that I was looking through dirty eye-glasses.

Some days my eyes appeared red around the edges of the top and bottom lids and dark circles appeared under my eyes. I found that using a white accent cream or applying more than one layer of makeup under the eyes lightened those dark circles.

There are no medical treatments available to prevent or treat these minor eye problems or relieve symptoms of distorted or cloudy vision. And their cause is unknown. Fortunately, they are temporary and will subside after the course of chemotherapy.

Only occasionally does more serious damage result from a com-bination of factors. These factors include the types and doses of chemotherapies, the overall condition of the patient and the condition of the eyes before chemotherapy. Sometimes the optic nerve, the retina, the cornea or the lens may be involved. The resulting changes may be temporary or permanent and cannot be predicted.

Safe Motoring

On days when my vision was cloudy, I was seriously concerned about driving safely. I feared that I might hit someone, especially on a gray day, and more especially if I needed to enter a dark parking garage. If I felt that I really needed to go someplace, I'd request a ride from a friend or family member.

I thought I was coping really well. Little did I know that there were more vision changes to come.

> *Now I can empathize with all those fish*
> *That swim around in their little glass dish.*
> *Looking through water is very strange*
> *I can hardly wait for my vision to change.*

Hot and Cold Flashes: Freezing and Frying

When estrogen is decreased in the body, spells of feeling hot followed by feeling cold often occur. During the course of chemotherapy, glandular function is usually suppressed. That includes the ovaries. Because some types of breast cancer are encouraged by estrogen, tamoxifen (Nolvadex) may be ordered to decrease the effects of natural estrogen. At the very least, estrogen replacement therapy is discontinued to discourage the growth of the breast cancer. Unfortunately, what is good for discouraging cancer growth is also good for fostering spells of feeling hot and cold.

Hot flashes come upon a woman without warning and may be potent. During a hot flash, off comes the sweater and off comes the wig, if the wearer is at home. Because so much heat is lost through the head, removing the wig speeds the cooling-off process and is a great relief.

However, hot flashes are more difficult to survive when not at home because not everyone wants to whip off the wig in public. During those moments, perspiration and fanning would be the keys to cooling off, except there is no perspiration! Those glands are suppressed so they don't function! So frantic fanning and frying are all that are left.

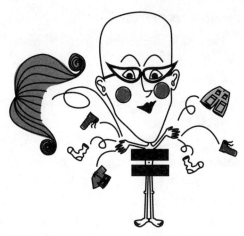

Hot flashes aren't so bad, as long as you're at home!

I have termed the spells of feeling cold as cold flashes. They are equally as uncomfortable and powerful. They usually follow the hot flashes and may be due to the cooling action of perspiration when those glands function. Cold flashes seem to penetrate to the very bone marrow. Teeth chatter and limbs shake. During these shaking chills, on goes the sweater, on goes the wig and maybe on goes a scarf around the neck to retain body heat.

Luckily, during a cold flash, having a wig to wear is wonderful. It's like wearing a fur hat. It's very effective in keeping heat in the body. Of course, that makes wearing a wig terribly uncomfortable on a hot summer day if the wearer is bothered by heat. But it helps during a cold flash.

Fortunately, flashes don't last very long and they may not occur everyday. But when they do, they are something. They can occur during the day or night. Obviously, at night, kicking off blankets goes a long way in relieving a hot flash, and whirling the knob to high on the electric blanket control helps to relieve the cold flash, although that is easier said than done in the midst of a shaking chill.

Some days seem like one round of off again, on again. Hot then cold, then hot then cold. Fortunately, these spells taper off and eventually go away. They don't last forever but they may last for several months after the cessation of chemo treatments. They just need to be weathered.

Feeling Normal

During a visit to my medical physician, I asked him about these dreadful cold flashes. Good soul that he is, he admitted that he'd never heard of this phenomenon. Of course, neither had I, even in my professional education and practice. Hot flashes, yes. But cold flashes, no.

I turned to my female friends and professional cohorts for information. Sure enough, I was not alone. Several of them had experienced the dreaded cold spells before or after their hot spells during estrogen withdrawal either during menopause or chemotherapy. I was much relieved! And even though I hated feeling cold with my limbs shaking and my teeth chattering, I learned that this was within the bounds of a normal reaction. So I stopped fretting about having some dreadful affliction in the vital centers of my brain.

There you have it. We can't expect physicians to know every little thing. Apparently, the freezing and frying cycles are not taught in medical school. Even postmenopausal male physicians cannot respond from their personal experience. They don't have the same symptoms as their female counterparts.

Quick Action Offsets a Hot Flash

Once when I was home and a hot flash was imminent, I whisked off my wig so fast that my eyeglasses flew across the floor. In my haste to head off the hot flash, I'd forgotten that I was wearing them. My only thought was to remove the article that caused me the most heat retention before the full impact of the flash hit me.

After cooling off a bit, I groped around to find my glasses. I finally retrieved them and placed them on my nose. When I regained my breath and opened my eyes, I discovered that my vision was very much out of focus. Oh, boy, I thought. Now what? I knew there could be vision changes, but to come on so suddenly was frightening to me. I tried to think of possible causes for this significant symptom. I logically deduced that the last hot flash might have fried my brain, or the ever-dreaded metastasis may have occurred or a super reaction to the chemotherapy could have transpired. I needed to think about this.

I moved along to the bathroom to sit a while and contemplate. The mirror caught my eye as I passed it and I halted my steps immediately. There was no reflection in my glasses—that meant no lenses in my glasses! So that's what caused my lack of focus.

Back to the livingroom I went and groped around some more. Sure enough, the lenses must have popped out when the glasses hit the floor. Lucky for me, they were intact and not even scratched. Such good fortune. In addition, my brain had not been fried. I should have bought a lottery ticket that day.

> First I'm hot and then I'm cold,
> I feel like I'm a sight to behold.
> I fan myself then I bundle up,
> I wonder if this will ever let up?

Fatigue: The Blahs

The blahs means that there is little energy for anything. That includes cooking, cleaning, caring for children and even getting out of bed in the morning. There is no energy for talking to friends or participating in social activities. It means that all one can think about is returning to bed and going to sleep or sitting in a chair and waiting for the return of vim and vigor. I could get up in the morning only because I knew I could return to bed whenever I felt tired. And nap I did—every single day. This was my most difficult symptom. I hated feeling "bone tired" all the time and dragging myself around.

I understood that the blahs signaled that the body was tired. It meant that the chemicals were working and sapping the body's energy. There was a war going on inside of me. It was the good guys (chemo drugs) against the bad guys (cancer cells). And I felt sidelined while this war was going on. I had to remind myself that those toxic chemo drugs affect every cell and system in the body. That's where my body's energy went. It was called survival on the cellular level, and I felt like a wet noodle because of it.

A drop in blood count can also cause fatigue. When the red cells decrease in number, the oxygen-carrying potential of the blood is diminished. Without the standard amount of oxygen, tiredness results. This drop in red blood cell count does not occur until after the second treatment and improves shortly after all the treatments are over, and maybe even before.

There are medications available on the market that can boost the red blood cell count so help is available.

For some unknown reason, some persons don't experience the blahs. Instead, they experience an increase in energy. This might be due to the steroid drugs administered before some chemotherapy agents. Some persons have enough energy to continue to work at their jobs throughout the course of treatment. Some need to have their work hours adjusted to meet the needs of chemo administration and their energy level.

Happily, having the blahs or having lots of energy is not a measure of how effectively the chemotherapy is working. The chemicals are doing the job either way.

To Work or Not to Work

Early in my course of treatment, I experienced big-time blahs. So, always seeking an excuse to pamper myself, I thought I had a good one in fighting cancer with chemo treatments—I retired from my job.

Because I happen to be a woman of a certain age, I was able to receive a retirement income. And I did just what I wanted to do. I kicked back in my recliner chair and pretended that I was queen for a day every day. I relaxed, read, munched, ran videos, watched TV and waited for the "cure."

Although I'm sure the time varies, it took 4 to 5 weeks after my last treatment for some steam to return to my engine. I felt the same as I did before the treatments except I was 1 or 2 pounds heavier. So all I needed was hair to be my old self.

> I'm just hanging around waiting for pep
> I hope it comes soon, I can't even schlep.
> I used to be out, going and doing
> Now I stay home with no energy brewing.

Other Facets in the Decision

I recognize that age does have its advantages. Because I was a woman of a certain age, I could retire. Not every woman has that choice, especially if it is the woman's job that provides the benefits for her family, especially health insurance.

There is a lovely young nurse who works at the emergency department of a local hospital who developed breast cancer. Because her job provided health insurance for her and her husband and young children, she needed to continue to work full time. Although she had sick time to cover her absence after the mastectomy, she returned to work, where she continued each day during her course of chemotherapy.

I think about her frequently. She was remarkable, with a positive attitude and expenditure of energy on the job. She must have been exhausted but she never complained. She just whizzed on her wig and went to work.

She had a great wig. People frequently complimented her on how becoming her new hairstyle was on her. She'd just smile and thank them. What a woman!

Looking back on my days of mothering three children and being a wife to a husband, I remember being tired at the end of the day. So I stand in awe of those women who just add chemotherapy to their otherwise busy days and keep on going.

Drop in Blood Count: The Count Crash

My chemotherapy was scheduled in 3-week cycles. So the most dangerous period for me within each cycle was from the seventh to the sixteenth days. On those days, I was particularly vulnerable to infection and bleeding because of my count crash. That means a low blood count. Vulnerable days vary according to the particular chemo drug being given.

Vulnerability occurs because chemotherapy depresses the bone marrow that makes red and white blood cells. White blood cells (WBCs) protect against infection. When they are in short supply, there is no defense against the invasion of disease-producing bacteria. Therefore, the body needs to be protected from exposure to all bacteria, including foreign bacteria, bacteria from the person's own body and bacteria from others.

Depending on the type of chemo, the number of white blood cells start dropping around the seventh day after each chemo administration. The lowest point for WBCs is usually from days 10 to 12 after administration of most breast cancer chemos. Then the count begins to come up, when cells are produced again. My WBCs were usually at their normal level by the twenty-first day, just in time for my next treatment in my 3-week cycle. Sometimes it takes a fourth week for the count to return to normal. If this is the case, the oncologist may postpone the chemotherapy one week or prescribe medication to increase the cell count.

To be safe during those vulnerable days, I tried to stay away from persons who were sick. I stayed away from crowds where colds might be rampant. I tried to be sure that persons who prepared my food and handled my dishes were not ill. When attending a group gathering where someone had a cold, I remained on the other side of the room, out of cough range.

I knew that it was important to wash my hands before and after doing anything, including eating, preparing food and using the bathroom. It was also important for the people who lived with me to do the same. I was careful to wash my hands after handling library books and items in stores. I used an antibacterial soap. I tried to keep my hands away from my face. I hadn't realized how often my hands went to my face before this effort. I tried to prevent cuts, burns and blisters. I used alcohol-free lotion to prevent drying my skin. I used tissues to blow my nose rather than my preferred hankie to avoid reintroduction of viruses into my nasal passages. Although this sounds like paranoia, it's really safety measures.

Red blood cells (RBCs) drop along with white blood cells but not as fast because red cells live longer than white cells. The red blood cells contain hemoglobin and hemoglobin carries oxygen. This drop in RBCs may not cause noticeable symptoms, but sometimes, when there is large decrease, a person may be short of breath and experience chest pain on exertion because of lack of oxygen in the circulating blood. In severe cases, a blood transfusion may be necessary. The physician should be notified if shortness of breath or chest pain occurs.

New medications have been developed to prevent or slow the drop in blood counts. Some help the body to increase blood counts. These drugs are not given preventatively but only when needed.

Contributing to My Retirement Decision

When I worked as a home care nurse, I often hiked up several flights of steps to visit homebound patients. I knew that with chemotherapy those days were at an end.

I knew that as my red blood cell count dropped, I would become too short of breath to reach those patients without presenting myself at the door gasping like a fish out of water. It made me chuckle to picture the expression on the faces of the patients and their caregivers when presented with a nurse who looked as though she herself was in need of resuscitation. I could not inflict that on those who have their own serious concerns.

Another Contribution to My Decision

An incident occurred that again prompted me to retire. This took me totally by surprise. It happened at the conclusion of my regular visit to one of my favorite senior female patients. She unexpectedly and suddenly expressed a genuine outpouring of affection for me. She made a fast grab at my head, got a hold of my hair, and pulled me toward her so she could give me a kiss on the cheek.

It was a heartfelt gesture that I really treasured. But once I recovered from the shock of this action, I realized that had I been wearing my wig, it might have come off in her hand or spun over my face during the aforementioned activity. That would have been such a shock for both of us that there might have been a real need for resuscitation. Although this imaginary scene gave me another chuckle, I would not have been laughing if it had really happened. Retirement was the right choice for me.

My white count is down, my red count is down,
And that darn flu bug is all over town.

Where can I hide? What can I do?
I'll stay home and avoid that flu.
When my bone marrow recovers I'll be ready to go
To find me you'll need to look high and low.
I'll be out on the town, 'cause I'll have endured,
I sure will be thankful when I am cured!

* * * * * *

I must be careful on those dangerous days,
And avoid unsafe practices in all ways.
Bacteria and viruses are everywhere
Of that dreadful fact I am well aware.
But they won't get me, they wouldn't dare
I know what to do and when to beware.

Fever: Hot Stuff

Several medications precede the administration of the chemo drugs through the vein. These medications minimize unpleasant side effects and help the recipient tolerate any that do occur. One is an antinausea medication to prevent nausea and vomiting. Another

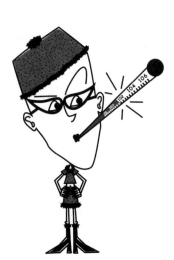

is a steroid medication that gives a feeling of well being but it also masks unpleasant symptoms that may occur from any cause, including those of an infection or cold. Most women do not acquire an infection during the course of chemotherapy because they have been well instructed and are careful.

An elevated temperature is one sign that the body has acquired an infection. In order to detect this, the oncologist may instruct the patient to take and record the morning temperature every day or at least on the days when the patient doesn't feel well.

Being 'hot stuff' wasn't all it was cracked up to be.

Chapter Six

When to Seek Emergency Care

By Joanna Brell, MD

Ask your oncologist about guidelines for going to the emergency room. Many doctors will want you to call them or their representative first; like you, they would prefer to handle a situation at home before necessitating a trip to the hospital. Your oncologist should have someone available by telephone 24 hours a day. Fever at the time when your white blood cell count is low is an emergency, but call your doctor first. Other major problems could include bleeding, shortness of breath or new-onset back pain, among others; call your doctor with symptoms as there are many possible scenarios for handling each problem.

If the body temperature rises above 100°F, instruction will be given as to what to do. Being "hot stuff" is not desirable during chemotherapy. Usually, the woman is told to go to the emergency room for treatment because this is a serious situation. The temperature is elevated because the immune system has been so depressed by the chemotherapy and the steroid drug that the body does not show severe symptoms like a high fever early in an illness. Thus when a slight elevation occurs, that person is already severely ill and treatment should be started as soon as possible.

It is a good idea to have the oncologist notified on arrival in the emergency room if not before leaving home. Treatment in the emergency room will begin quickly. These measures will help fight the infection wherever it is in the body.

Keeping Track

I kept a calendar in the bathroom where I took my temperature every morning on arising and recorded it along with other symptoms I experienced. My plan was to be very careful and avoid an infection or a cold. By now, I felt like I was keeping the medical community going single-handedly, and I was tired of it. And I was a member of that community!

Though life is a gamble every day,
Fever is a symptom with which I won't play.
For this is a signal however weak
That indicates medical attention to seek.
And even though I don't feel bad
I'll go to the ER and leave my pad.
Treatment will help me and then I'll be
Ready for more chemotherapy.

Headache: A Thumper

A real thumper of a headache can develop during administration of chemotherapy or at any time during the next 24 hours. This is often a monster headache with throbbing, pulsating pain.

If the headache occurs during administration, it may mean that the chemical agent is being given more rapidly than the person can tolerate. Or it may mean that one of the medications is at fault. Slowing the infusion rate often relieves the headache.

If it occurs after administration, whatever usually works to relieve a headache will probably work. Taking Tylenol or acetaminophen can be effective. Rest also helps. Taking aspirin during the course of treatment is not recommended because aspirin encourages bleeding when the platelet count is below normal.

Making Adjustments

The worst headaches I experienced during chemotherapy were those caused by the combination of my eyeglasses and wig.

After my experience of chasing my wig across the parking lot, I considered all factors to try to fit it snugly on my head. I placed the temples of my glasses outside the wig and arranged the hair over them. I counted on those temples to help anchor the wig. This seemed to be a workable arrangement.

I finally learned that wigs have an adjustable mechanism along the bottom edge and across the back up to the ear tabs. That mechanism is what caused the problem because it got in the way of the temples on my glasses. Behind my ears, the tip of the temples sat directly on top of that triple-layered cloth tape mechanism with its Velcro closure. That was the source of my headaches! Pressure, pain and agony, and almost two holes in my head!

Although I went out and about with my wig in place, I had to wear my glasses if I wanted to see where I was going. But I couldn't stay out too long without developing a headache. So those were quick trips. When home again, I quickly exchanged the wig for a turban and placed the temples inside. There you have it! My secrets of success to relieve pressure and avoid headaches.

> *What's with my head, it sometimes thumps,*
> *Causing me to be down in the dumps.*
> *I hate headaches, they incapacitate me*
> *They pound on my brain till I can hardly see.*
> *They may not last long and they're not truly rife,*
> *They're just another bump on the road of life.*

Maintaining Relationships

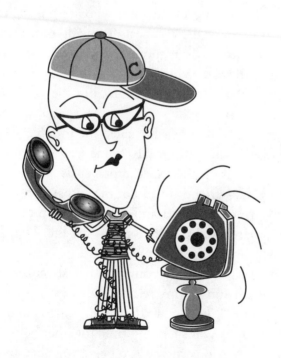

L ife after surgery and during chemotherapy can be stressful on relationships. First, the patient has little energy and a great need to rest and sleep. A certain degree of depression may occur and a desire of folding in on yourself to heal in isolation rather than socialize, especially with those who have not been through the same experience.

Second, visitors expect a certain amount of cheeriness in the person they are visiting and that takes a lot of energy. Some visitors stay too long and that can be exhausting. But visitors are to be treasured because they truly care or they wouldn't have made the effort to come.

If the patient is young, has a mate or significant other, children and a job, most energy will need to go there. So in-person socialization with friends can take away from that energy pool. However, a card or a quick phone call is priceless and treasured.

There are many volunteers out there who are waiting to help those who need it. Some deliver meals, some do grocery shopping, some drive persons to medical appointments and some come into the home to give the caregiving family a respite. Some volunteers you may know, some you may not know, but they all have the desire to serve those in need.

I was amazed at the friends who called me to offer their assistance with transportation and meals. Some just wanted to say hello and tell me that I was on their special prayer list. Some I had not heard from in years—friends from out of my past who wanted to be of help. It warmed my heart and cheered me up to know that these people were ready and able to rejoin my life. They lifted my spirits and I will always be grateful.

One positive result from my bout with breast cancer and surgeries was the strengthening of my relationship with my children. I never felt so treasured. I guess we didn't talk much about life, love, gratefulness and the joy of spending time together before my illness. Now we do. We look forward to being together and sharing our lives in a more meaningful way. What a wonderful support they were to me during that difficult time.

Sexuality

I found it strange to look in the mirror and see only one breast and an unflattering new incision. Of course, when the incision healed and the stitches and drainage tubes had been removed, the incision faded. But lack of symmetry yields an unbalanced appearance and arouses feelings of being a undesirable feminine persona.

In my case, I was not married. However, I thought that my appearance would not inspire feelings of desirability from any possible candidate. I could not imagine seeking a new husband after my mastectomy. I did not feel very sensuous or lust provoking.

But my experience with married couples has been positive. The patients' loved ones have been supportive and thoughtful, sometimes going out of their way to make the women feel cared for and appreciated.

Communication about feelings and expectations is important. Issues about cuddling and resuming intercourse after the surgery and during chemotherapy are important topics to talk about even when healthy. Not everyone is at his or her peak when intercourse is suggested. Certainly, common sense would dictate that when one partner is vomiting is not the best time to suggest it.

In addition to physical appearance, exhaustion may contribute to the lack of interest in sex. If the woman has the responsibility of small children, a job and housework, it may be hard to find the energy for a lustful frolic. Sexual appetite may be as suppressed as the appetite for food. This will improve as treatments continue. But partners talking to each other about this is a big step in the right direction.

Sex

A friend of mine was determined to keep a fully functional sex life with her husband during chemotherapy. Because the function of all glands in the body is suppressed, she knew that the glands that lubricate the vaginal canal would also be affected. So she headed this problem off at the pass by buying some KY Jelly to insert before the act was under way.

The Question of Intimacy

By Barbara Tripp, RN

The issue of intimacy is very complex. For some women, this will be the most difficult area of adjustment. Perhaps the best way to start is to differentiate the physical issues from the emotional ones. Pain and the more lasting sensitivity of the surgical area, fatigue, nausea, vomiting, body aches and all the other possible side effects of treatment you may experience will interfere with your desire and enjoyment of being close to even the one you care most about. These problems should be temporary. Talking with your doctor and/or nurse may also help you find ways to minimize the problems.

The more difficult issues are related to the emotional aspects of intimacy. A lot depends on the strength of the relationship before the diagnosis of breast cancer. Identifying the strengths and weaknesses of the relationship is essential to dealing with questions and concerns during this period of adjustment. Many couples will work through these new ups and downs as they have worked through previous life stresses. They may find their relationship to be even stronger. Other couples will need the help of professional counseling to survive.

If you are not in a relationship at the time of diagnosis, you may be dealing with the uncertainty of how you will cope with this issue in the future. Think of it as an additional aspect of the "getting to know you" phase of any new relationship and how much it will reveal about the other person's character. Key to dealing with others is how you perceive yourself. This is an ongoing, lifelong, ever-evolving process for everyone. As we become stronger as individuals, our relationship with others will benefit.

She knew one night that sex was imminent. Unbeknownst to her husband, she slipped into the bathroom and gave the KY Jelly tube a serious squeeze, depositing the lubricating gel into the vagina. Then she had to hurry to bed because as the gel warmed, it began to run down her leg.

Although her husband was anxious about the first relationship after chemo began, he was surprised and delighted at the ease of the process. Insertion was smooth, the path well lubricated. He commented that she had an abundance of lubrication like she had when she was younger when they first married. He attributed that to the chemo and, in a way, the chemo was directly responsible. She was pleased that his path was made easier and never mentioned that she lay in a gel puddle all night. But the next time, she paved the way with a little less gel in that strategic location.

Communication

Man is a social being and so are the women who are receiving chemotherapy for treatment of breast cancer. Each person has her own way of dealing with illness and treatment. Some desire the ultimate privacy and want to be silent about it. Some find it is easier to live with it if they share this information. Some seek the assistance of others who have been down the same road of diagnosis, surgery and chemo. Support groups are especially good for them. Most cancer centers have counselors available for sharing the various approaches to this task.

Women with husbands and children have unique needs and may seek special support systems. Telling these family members can be very difficult. But the results can be especially gratifying because those relationships can become so much stronger.

My Communication Mistake

The day I went to the surgeon's office, he examined the lump, biopsied it, sent it to pathology but declared there was no doubt in his mind that it was cancer. So we scheduled surgery for the following week, the first available opportunity.

My plan was to inform my children first but I was afraid of that conversation. I was sure that I would blubber during the conversation about this happening and I didn't want to boo hoo through it. So I very carefully wrote a note to each of them and mailed them off to the East Coast where they all live. I felt relieved.

That turned out to be a disaster. I should have told them in person or at least with my own voice. They were so upset at opening a note from me and discover that their mother had cancer and was already scheduled for surgery. They were stunned by the news and felt disconnected when they were not able to immediately reach me by phone. All kinds of questions swirled around in their heads, none of which they could ask or get answered. My method of communicating this important information was a big mistake and I do not recommend it. I was thinking of making the process easier on myself, and gave no thought to the folks on the receiving end.

The Big Secret

After I spoke with my children, I decided to tell only immediate family members and a few close friends of my diagnosis and treatment plan. I wanted it to be our secret. I did not want it discussed all over town. I was a very private person about my personal health matters. I had not intended to tell the world, especially mere acquaintances.

Imagine my surprise when I received a card from the Sunshine Committee of a volunteer group I occasionally attended! Then came a phone call from the president of that organization who assured me that all members of the group would be praying for my recovery. I practically fainted dead away! I was speechless and infuriated! I had told a friend, who told a friend, and that friend is one Chatty Cathy. I should have known better! I should have realized that the news might reach Chatty Cathy, who never keeps anything to herself.

The lesson I learned was that once anyone was told something, it was no longer a secret. The word was out. I needed to let go of my anger and the idea of keeping this secret. I needed to adjust myself to the fact that the news was out on the drums and I couldn't control it.

In the long run, I found that it was comforting to share the diagnosis and treatment with family members, close friends and coworkers. I benefited from it and our relationships have grown stronger. I was surprised at the number of friends who asked about helping me, driving me places and shopping for me. It was gratifying to know that people wanted to help me. I realized that people who wanted to be helpful needed someone to help. And by allowing that help we served each other's needs.

Communication Guidelines

By Barbara Tripp, RN

Trust is a key element in a healthy relationship. Without honesty, trust is jeopardized. Decisions about whom to tell about your diagnosis, and what or how much to tell may take some thought. Sometimes, the first impulse is not to tell a particular person. Family members who are very old or very young (refer to books on dealing with the special needs of children in Appendix C) are often shielded from information. This is done for many reasons. To shield means to protect. But think hard about what is being protected. Who is being protected? What benefit will the protection provide? To not tell someone about your diagnosis or to share the information in code, that is, to not use the word *cancer* or to underestimate or sugarcoat the reality of the situation, may be at the very least confusing, and perhaps even, in some cases, perceived as a betrayal.

The following are guidelines in communicating:

- Be truthful! Avoid making false assurances.

- Be timely. Once you've told one person, news travels fast. Communicating in a timely manner avoids misconceptions and someone hearing from an inappropriate source.

- Be kind. Anger can sometimes get in the way when communicating difficult news. Being brutal or too blunt can be cruel.

- Use age- and situation-appropriate terms. Information should be clear and understood but need not be explicit.

- If you are unable to give information yourself, especially if you have a large family or group of friends, choose an appropriate alternate. This may be especially helpful if the treatment will be lengthy.

In the long run, I decided to tell the world. So I wrote this book. In my illustrious past, I had been a teacher of patients and nursing students. And that becomes a way of life. I decided that because the information I sought about the side effects of chemotherapy was not readily available, I found there to be a need for this book.

Partners

I don't have a husband or significant other so I am not the best person to make suggestions in this category. But I have friends and relatives who do have mates who care about them greatly and I see what a special support they can be.

A loving partner can be priceless in emotional help to the woman and a true help with the work in running a household. When children are involved, the partner can be the leader of the support team, to appreciate the woman and mom and do special chores to relieve her. The partner can take the children to the park or zoo to let the mom get some extra rest, especially the first few days after the chemo treatment when she is particularly tired, and cook a few dinners or carry out or carry in on other days. If the mom is nauseated, she may not even be able to approach the kitchen. So it may fall to the partner to do the grocery shopping, cooking and cleanup so the patient is away from even the odors of food.

The strengthening of a partnership can be the best thing about this horrible situation. When a catastrophe like cancer occurs in a life, many things are thought about and appreciated that may have been overlooked or taken for granted before the calamity. Adversity can bring partners together so that they will be closer than they ever would have been without the disaster that has befallen them.

Weathering the cancer crisis together and being supportive of each other is a valuable goal in this situation and one that will never be forgotten by either party. If children are involved, this incidence will not be easy but will bring the family closer together. We learn to treasure each other when we are afraid of loss.

Of course, every day will not be a joyous day of lovey-dovey and cozying. Emotions run high inside of everyone in the home. Laughter, sorrow, anger, happiness, children acting out in a negative way, short tempers are all a part of life. And cancer, chemo, exhaustion and disbelief in the whole scenario are all a part of life with cancer and its treatment.

But hang in there. It will get better as time and communication go on. The aftereffects of chemotherapy will go away and you will be back to your old self and have better and stronger relationships than ever before.

Children

Children's needs vary according to their age. But at any age, children feel threatened and get upset when told that their mother has cancer. There are several good books on the market that can be used to explain cancer and its treatment to little children. These are listed in Appendix C.

Children will be affected. My niece's 7-year-old son went up to his teacher every school morning for about eight weeks to announce to her that his mother had cancer. The teacher knew that this child needed to share this information so he could go on with his day. So the teacher referred him to the school counselor. Now he says that he has an adult friend with whom he talks and can say anything to. This counseling has proven to be a big help to this little guy.

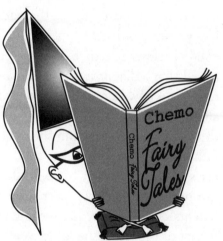

It's not easy explaining chemo to your kids, even when they are adults.

Now he seems able to accept the scenario and has stopped announcing this cancer problem to his teacher every day. He has made a good adjustment.

A mother who is going off to surgery or who is experiencing the aftereffects of chemo affects children of all ages. The last thing I remember as I was wheeled to surgery for the mastectomy was my oldest daughter crying her eyes out. She was in her 30s but deeply felt some of the situations that she and I might be facing in the future.

Little ones cannot be shielded from every symptom. Sometimes children might see their mother vomiting into the toilet and that might be frightening. The loss of hair is certainly a change in the mother's appearance and needs discussion and reassurance.

This is one situation that is a family experience. Each member of the family is affected in his or her own way. Sometimes counseling can be helpful to bring out feelings and assist each family member to cope.

Parents

Breast cancer, or any cancer, is also hard on parents, who are usually not prepared to see their adult children in pain. However, like so many of life's crises, serious illness can bring parents and children closer together. This happened to my friend Lisa who found that a diagnosis of breast cancer at age 29 gave her a chance to get to know her mother better. Lisa quickly discovered that of all of the people who stood by her during that time, her mom was the "one true rock" whom she could always depend on. From day 1, her mother never left her side, accompanying her to the radiologist's office, staying by her bedside after surgery and being with her during chemotherapy. After surgery, Lisa chose to recover at her parents' home, where her mom gave her special care and even fed her all of the treats she loved as a kid— ice cream, soda and popsicles. Even though chemo treatment isn't one of the most pleasurable things, Lisa's mom helped lighten the load and made the experience into a special routine by stopping for lunch on the way home from her work. Although Lisa may not have been able to stomach everything on her plate those days, she treasures the enjoyable conversations she and her mom shared as they sat through their lunches!

Extended Family

Who and how to tell family members is a personal choice. In some cases, the patient wants to personally deliver the news; in other cases, a daughter or friend may be selected to pass along the information.

It is amazing how many people are out there waiting to do something for someone. It helps them to know of someone they can help, especially a family member.

My niece designed a Web site for all who are interested in keeping up with her progress. That has really simplified her life. So she writes one note on the Web site as her condition changes and all interested parties can tune in and get it. And they do—family members, friends and coworkers.

It's an imaginative Web site. Because she is a big fan of the Cleveland Indians baseball team, she placed a large stick figure wearing a Cleveland Indian baseball cap on her Web site. And because it is an interactive Web site, you can read a message from her, and leave a message for her. You can also leave a message or a joke for any of her three children, who have their separate icons as well.

Sometimes she has something we Web site visitors can vote for, such as, should she wear a wig or a hat on her bare head. There is a running tally so you can keep track of the public's opinion.

This is such a fresh and fun way to communicate. It makes us laugh at the little jokes and asides she notes in her messages to her fans. It makes us want to be a part of her life and lift her spirits. And, in turn, she lifts ours.

Friends

Friends are true treasures. They come through with positive thoughts, cards, phone calls, visits and in a hundred other much appreciated ways. There is nothing like them. They might be neighbors, schoolmates or church or club mates. It is remarkable how they just show up when they are needed. Sometimes they gather together to make a plan to help.

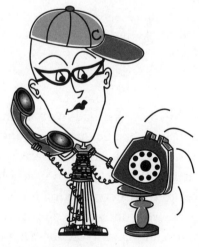

Speed dial was a necessity.

Accepting Help from Friends

By Barbara Tripp, RN

Friends are a valuable resource! If a friend offers you help, stop and think before responding. Sometimes we are too quick to answer and too often thank the person for offering but decline the help. We may be too indoctrinated in "it is better to give than to receive."

Accepting help may be difficult. Be creative in coming up with ways people can help. Helping with shopping, cooking, transporting, providing lawn care, finding a cleaning service, watching children while you sneak in a nap, or even appointing someone to assign others helpful tasks may be invaluable in getting through the tough times.

Most of us can use help even in less stressful, less hectic times. If the offer is genuine, the person will feel good that they are able to help. You can help them to feel good. Accepting help can put a positive spin on what is otherwise a new and/or uncomfortable behavior.

Others may disappoint you. The person you most expect to be there for you, may be nowhere to be found. Some people simply cannot face illness, cannot be near it.

Communication and patience are important in any relationship. Many women find that their priorities change and their needs and wants take on new dimensions. Honesty is always a good policy. Learning the fine art of being kind and gentle, yet telling it like it is may help you and others during this difficult and trying time.

Not everyone will attempt to understand what you are going through. Reaching out when in need while learning to set limits and boundaries may help in striking the balance of support and privacy.

My niece has had many positive experiences with friends during her siege. She belongs to a book club with fourteen members. When she told them she was going to have breast surgery and chemo, they decided to have a hat party. Each woman brought a hat to their next meeting for Maureen to wear. Some were stylish, some were outrageous, some were just plain funny and some were warm and cozy. Now she has a closet full of fun and fancy hats, and her 2-year-old daughter helps her select which hat she should wear if she's not going to wear her wig, which Carolyn has named the "hair hat." It's a big mother-daughter thing—another special connection and another reason to be merry.

Members of Maureen's church organized a Bring-a-Dinner program. Every night for one week after each of Maureen's chemo treatments, the person who volunteered for that evening, brings dinner to the house. Because Maureen will receive eight treatments (3 weeks apart), that amounts to fifty-six dinners that will be delivered. Then during the 6 weeks of radiation, dinner will be provided every night. That's another forty-two dinners.

This has created quite a spirited fun and imaginative contest kind of feeling among the group in order that there is not a lot of repetition and to gain a reputation. One gentleman called to take their order for a Chinese dinner that he was going to call in and carry out to them. Some plan and cook special dinners in their homes and then deliver them.

On the night before her first chemo, some friends pooled their money and had a romantic gourmet dinner for two delivered from an elegant restaurant. Not only was the food delivered, but the wine, white linen tablecloth, silverware and candles came along too. Maureen and her husband, Dave, did not think about chemotherapy that night.

Some members of Dave's union wanted to do something for Dave and his fine family of five. So they collected enough money to buy an upright freezer for them, something that the couple had been saving for over time. What an outpouring of friendship and camaraderie has been expressed toward this lovely family! What a difference in their stress level to have such a broad level of support!

Organizations

Many persons who have had cancer seek organizations to share their thoughts and feelings with others. These organizations can be helpful to boost the spirits of the members and to learn about how to cope with various symptoms.

Finding a Support Group

By Barbara Tripp, RN

Some ideas that may be helpful when searching for support include

- Church groups, even if not a member; women's circles, men's clubs, mission committees may all be willing to offer anything, from financial assistance to meals or transportation; ministers, priests, rabbis, Stephen ministers, etc., are a potential source of individuals who are available to listen, counsel or provide spiritual guidance.

- Wellness communities available locally, nationally, or on-line (computers may be available at the hospital or the local library if you do not own one).

- Schools and PTAs often rally and provide meals; fundraisers; counseling for children whose parent, grandparent, aunt or sister is dealing with breast cancer; they also may provide a space in which to start a support group.

- Service-oriented community groups such as Kiwanis, Rotary Club, Key Club, Junior Achievement, Girl or Boy Scout troops, etc.

- Cities and towns may have a Department of Human Services (or at least an individual) available to provide phone calls to someone living alone, transportation to a doctor's appointment, or tips on individuals or groups in the community who may lend assistance.

- Employers may have an Employee Assistance Program (EAP) that are knowledgeable on community resources and/or provide counseling to the employee and, sometimes, the employee's family.

Selecting a Support Team

Every person needs a support team; that is, the persons who will help with day-to-day living, such as shopping, cleaning, child sitting, cooking, arranging family activities, and serve as a confidant. Of course, the woman's husband or partner is often the biggest support system but because of probably also working full time, the husband or partner cannot fulfill all the roles that will be needed.

Husbands and partners also need support teams, friendship and lots of compliments and hugs. Ask him or her how they are doing from time to time, and listen to their tales. Ask how all of this is affecting his or her life. So often the partner or husband is deep in the shadows because all the attention is going to the woman. They need some attention, love and support as well.

Confidant

Not everyone is interested or comfortable in sharing their lives with a group. Some are not available at the specific time a group meets. Sometimes, choosing a friend or neighbor who has been through the chemotherapy process can serve as a mentor for questions and advice. This may be a less stressful way to share thoughts and feelings. Developing a close relationship with one mature experienced person may be the direction to take for some women.

Decisions

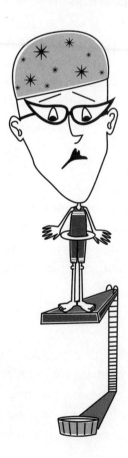

A situation in which cancer is involved requires several serious decisions. The overall treatment plan is one of them. Would it be best to begin with some radiation treatments to shrink the tumor and then have surgery? Should a lumpectomy or mastectomy be the surgery of choice? Would it be best to have chemotherapy or radiation, or both? What kind of chemo would be most effective?

These decisions will be made with guidance and knowledge of the surgeon and oncologist. They can guide your decision-making but often you have the final say. These decisions will affect the rest of your life as well as the quality of that life.

Type of Surgery

The type of surgery performed may not be completely the patient's decision. Certainly, the surgeon will explain all the possible options, but some decisions must be made in the operating room according to findings as the surgery proceeds.

Much depends on the location and size of the tumor, the type of cancer cells, the lymph node involvement and the patient's decision about having reconstructive surgery.

Chemotherapy

Upon discussing the pros and cons of various chemotherapies that could be effective, the oncologist often gives the woman the final choice. There may be more than one kind of chemo that might be capable of arresting the cancer growth but one might be slightly better than the another. That is where a decision must be made.

Employment

To work or not to work during weeks of chemotherapy—that is the question. I had the opportunity to retire and was happy for it.

But retirement is not an option for some women. They may not be of retirement age. Their income may be needed to support the family. They may need to work for the medical insurance benefits.

Choosing a Treatment

By Joanna Brell, MD

Cancer continues to be studied by scientists and doctors; all information known today comes from laboratory experiments, clinical trials and documentation before us. Each type of cancer (i.e., adenocarcinoma of the breast, lymphoma, squamous cell carcinoma of the lung, melanoma, etc.) has been deliberately tested with many types of treatments. The treatments with the best success rate are often used first. Sometimes there are two or more types of chemotherapies that can be used and your doctor can explain the risks, benefits and alternatives of each one. For breast carcinoma, other factors such as the tumor grade, size of tumor, number of lymph nodes and hormone receptor status can be used to determine your chemotherapy plan. These decisions are extremely complex and you will need to ask questions until you understand why a certain therapy is best in your situation. Remember, there are times when it's best to take a lesser treatment because it has fewer side effects that could potentially be harmful. Clinical trials are available continually and could be an excellent way to obtain state-of-the-art therapy.

I know many nurses who work full time during their course of treatment. Wearing a wig and a smile on their face, they are on the job ministering to the patients who need their help. They need to be careful of persons who have a contagious condition so their coworkers usually take on those patients. If necessary, they can wear a face mask to protect themselves from respiratory conditions. They may be able to have their chemotherapy administered at the end of a workday, then schedule their two days off following that to give them time to recover. If their blood count drops in mid cycle between chemo sessions, they may need to take a few sick days until the count rebounds.

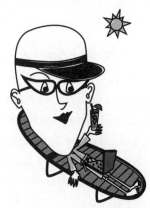

Working from home was a great option.

Radiation

By Joanna Brell, MD

Radiation therapy can be used with or without chemotherapy or hormonal therapy for breast carcinoma. This type of treatment is localized and affects only where the x-ray beam is pointed; therefore, the entire body is not influenced. If one has had a lumpectomy, radiation therapy is mandatory to prevent the cancer from returning to the same breast. If you don't want radiation, then you must have a mastectomy. It is now known that some women who have had a full mastectomy benefit from radiation therapy. If the tumor was large in size (i.e., around 4 cm or more), involved many lymph nodes (usually four or more) or adhered to the tissues of the chest, then radiation can further decrease the risk of recurrence to the chest wall. Usually radiation therapy is given after surgery and chemotherapy; you will need to be assessed by a specially trained radiation oncologist.

Working full time is not easy during chemotherapy. Other options may be investigated before the decision is made. It may be possible to drop to part time during the treatment period. It may be possible to connect with the office by computer and work at home some of the time. Whatever work schedule is determined, rest is an all-important factor in recovering from the chemo treatments. To become weak and run-down can invite a cold or infection and complicate the treatment and endanger the patient's life.

Focusing Energy

I found that during the morning hours until after an early lunch was my peak time for energy level and productive projects. After lunch, I faded away and was delighted to climb into bed for a delicious nap. Because I live alone and am not responsible for little children or have a husband to care for, I could snooze as long as I chose. Although aloneness has a downside, it has its rewards as well.

Working full time, being responsible for small children and maintaining a relationship with a loving husband sounds like three full-time jobs to me. Establishing a specific time to rest and nap is essential in this setting. Here is when family members, friends, parents of the children's playmates and neighbors can help.

Complementary Therapies

There are several complementary therapies that proclaim value in their use in the treatment of cancer and can be used as supplementary therapy. Principal among them are dietary alterations, macrobiotics, use of herbs, lifestyle modifications, exercise therapy, hydrotherapy, aromatherapy, T'ai chi and acupuncture. Other choices include biofeedback, visualization, meditation, hypnosis, yoga, Reiki, nutritional supplements and vitamins. It is always a good idea to check with the oncologist to be sure that the selection

Alternative and Complementary Therapies

By Joanna Brell, MD

Alternative therapies are usually thought of as unproven treatments; if they have been tested and found to be helpful, then they are classified as traditional therapies. In this light, all new potential treatments start as alternative therapies. Unfortunately, many developers of alternative treatments will not submit their ideas for research, leaving your doctor without any scientific information to share with you. Given the options of using a proven treatment with known side effects versus an alternative therapy known only by word of mouth, most doctors will recommend the established treatment. Natural substances cannot promise fewer adverse effects, as many medications and chemotherapies are derived from plants. Scientific testing is the only way to get valid information on these substances.

Complementary therapies are considered to be additional treatments that are applied with conventional treatment. Again, not all of these have been scientifically assessed, and there are no claims of killing cancer cells; these therapies are not used for that purpose. Also, interactions between these and standard therapies are largely unknown, but in general they are not thought to be harmful. They are considered to assist one as they go through traditional therapy, such as massage, acupuncture, relaxation, vitamins, etc. Always discuss everything you are doing with your doctor.

of a supplementary therapy is consistent with the treatment regimen. A conflict there would not be helpful.

Because I am a conventional person, I moved immediately toward traditional medicine and proven treatments. I have added some others along the way, such as a multivitamin and the herb, Echinacea—to build up my immune system and prevent colds and infections. Although I stuck pretty close to the conventional paths, there is a lot to be said for integrating the complementary therapies. More complementary therapies are described in Appendix E.

Follow-Up Care

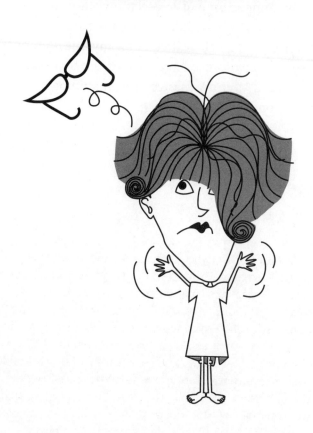

A fter surgery, each patient is scheduled to return to the surgeon's office for checkups to be sure the incision has healed and the cancer has not returned. The same is true after chemotherapy. Each patient must return to the oncologist for examinations to see that the cancer has not returned to the opposite breast or to the operated breast. Although individual physicians may differ a little in scheduling visits, the oncologist follows each patient at least annually for the patient's lifetime.

Check with the oncologist regarding the odds of recurrence concerning each particular kind of cancer. This will vary with the type of cancer, the extent of invasion and location of the original site.

Physician Visits

Visits to the lumpectomy or mastectomy surgeon vary with the surgeon. My visits were scheduled every 6 months for the first 2 years, then once per year thereafter. After my lumpectomy, mammograms were ordered every 6 months for the first year then one per year after that. After my mastectomy, mammograms were scheduled only once per year.

Follow-Up Visits

By Joanna Brell, MD

In checking for metastatic disease, other medical conditions can be found. Metastatic breast cancer often goes to the liver, lungs and bones, so these areas are inspected by asking the patient specific questions, by physical examination and by x-rays. Regularly, these studies reveal arthritic changes of the bone, which may look like cancer on a bone scan and which would require further x-rays to differentiate. Cysts of the liver and benign tumors, including tangles of blood vessels, may be noted, which are usually of no consequence. One may also have benign tumors of the lung, scars from old infections and emphysema seen on lung x-rays. None of these things is related to breast cancer. No radiographic studies need to be repeated unless a new problem, such as pain, develops.

I did not need to visit the plastic surgeon after I had the final reconstructive surgery and was healed. That was good news to me. I could scratch one off the appointment docket.

Visits to my oncologist were scheduled every 3 months for the first 2 years, then every 6 months for 3 years and once a year thereafter.

Some oncologists include blood tests and x-rays as a part of the follow-up exams. Some do not because of the possibility of incomplete information and unnecessary worry.

A blood test may be done to check for liver enzymes. If they are within normal range the liver is functioning well. If not, liver metastasis is suspected and further tests may be ordered.

A chest x-ray is done to determine if the cancer has spread to the lungs. Special x-rays can be done to study bones. Often, it is pain that indicates that bone metastasis has occurred.

Sometimes suspicious lesions appear on x-rays and mammograms that are not cancerous. There are many abnormal conditions that can afflict a person and yet the body can function normally. Not every shadow on a diagnostic test is a malignancy.

My Big Scare

Before beginning chemotherapy, my oncologist requested a chest x-ray to determine the condition of my lungs and a CAT scan of my liver to determine if there was metastasis there. When I returned to her office to get the reports, she said that she had some news that was not very good.

She showed me my chest x-ray and the bones were spotted all over with white blotches. When she showed me the liver picture, she pointed out two separate dark spots that were each about the size of a dime.

She said that there should be further tests done to see if these spots were cancers, because if they were, I had between 1 and 2 years to live. It also would make a difference in my chemo treatment plan.

So a special x-ray of my chest bones and an ultrasound of my liver were scheduled. I was praying hard. After the results were in, I returned to meet with my oncologist once again. She greeted me with a big hug. Both tests were negative. They turned out to be false-positives. The spots on my ribs were arthritis and the spots on my liver were cysts. Was I happy! What a relief! What a special day!

Scaring a Doctor

During the preoperative screening before the surgical insertion of my permanent prosthesis, the medical physician performed a check of my reflexes and other neurological tests. I followed his finger back and forth while he watched to see that my eyes could follow. I looked up, down and side to side.

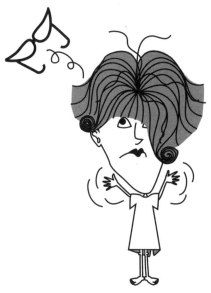

Then he asked me to raise my eyebrows to see if they moved evenly. When I did that, my penciled in brows disappeared up under the bangs of my wig. I hadn't realized but in the course of raising myself up and down on the examining table, my wig had slipped forward, the tip of the bangs almost touching the bridge of my nose.

Try not to scare your doctors.

When the doctor couldn't visualize my eyebrows, he began to struggle with my bangs so he could see more clearly. Embarrassed, I reached up, grabbed hold of the crown of the wig and moved the whole thing back, positioning it more properly on my head. He didn't say anything but he didn't keel over and land on the floor at my feet either. That was the end of the exam. I think he lost his concentration on neurological testing.

Breast Self-Exam

Breast self-exam continues to top the list of important steps in discovering early breast cancer. That is because more women find

Breast Cysts

By Joanna Brell, MD

Many women have cysts in their breasts; you could have just a few, or your breasts could be packed with cysts. Breast tissue expands and contracts in response to natural hormones, beginning at puberty; it is normal to develop cysts in areas of such constant change. When examining your breasts, you do not have to decide if a lump is a cyst or cancer. However, you have to determine if it is a change from the way your breasts usually feel; if it is, notify your doctor.

their own lumps than lumps detected on mammograms. There's not much of an excuse for not doing it. Your breasts are with you all the time. It's not that you can't find a place to park.

The monthly manual exam of the entire breast is really important. You know your own breasts, know how they hang, what they feel like and where the usual lumps are located. And it doesn't take much time. You can do it when you go to bed at night or before you get up in the morning or in the shower when you're soaped up.

The most frequent sites of cancer are the areas around and under the nipple and the upper outer quadrant of each breast. These areas should be carefully examined and changes reported to the physician.

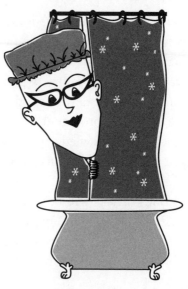

More lumps are discovered by women doing self-exams than by mammograms.

On the mastectomy or lumpectomy side, the areas under and around the incision are the most likely areas to develop a cancerous growth. Even after a mastectomy, cancer can recur. It is almost impossible to remove every single breast cell because breast tissue is integrated into the skin. So be on the lookout for recurrences, especially in those sites.

A Repeat Performance

After my lumpectomy, the cancer returned along the incision line. My surgeon called it an extension of the original tumor. My oncologist called it a recurrence. I wanted neither one, but if I had to make a choice, I'd take the extension. I did not want to consider any stray cancer cells floating around in my body, lodging anywhere, even in the same breast. I found it interesting that each physician expressed a different opinion and both were adamant in their appraisals. Oh well, mastectomy time!

Mammogram

It will continue to be important to have a mammogram once a year following the removal of a breast cancer. Because 30 million mammograms are done every year in the United States, most radiologists are getting pretty good at reading them. In fact, there are some radiologists who specialize in reading mammograms. They are especially proficient in detecting breast cancer. An up-to-date machine, a knowledgeable and careful technologist and a radiologist who reads many mammograms help to improve the accuracy of the procedure.

Both breasts will be x-rayed if a lumpectomy was done.

If you have had a mastectomy, only the remaining breast will be x-rayed, even if you have had a prosthesis implanted. A manual exam will need to suffice on the mastectomy side.

Looking for a Bargain

After my mastectomy and reconstruction, I was told that a mammogram would be performed on both breasts because cancer can recur on the side of the mastectomy. I wondered how that would be possible on the mastectomy side. I certainly didn't want the prosthesis to explode under the pressure of the x-ray machine. I was assured that the prosthesis was strong and that it would not explode.

When I arrived at the radiology department, I was informed that a mammogram would not be done on the mastectomy side. That was a relief! I didn't favor returning to surgery to replace a blown-up balloon.

After my one-sided mammogram was done, I thought about contacting both the billing department and the radiologist to ask if the procedure and the reading would be half price because only one breast had been x-rayed. Unfortunately, I could not bring myself to do that. It just didn't seem professional. But I really wanted to know.

Next I tried to compare the price of my one-sided postoperative mammogram to my two-sided preoperative mammogram. But price comparison was too difficult using insurance papers. Charges and negotiated fees change too rapidly. Also, I couldn't compare with previous insurance papers because I had prior mammograms done in a different facility. Finally, the question about the price was answered for me by calling the billing department of the hospital anonymously. The answer is it costs less than a double mammogram but more than a single mammogram. Depending on the facility and radiologist, it costs about one-and-one-half the price of a single mammogram.

10

The Future

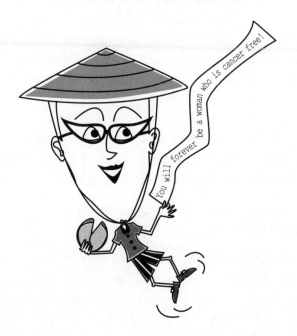

God only knows
What the future holds.
But I have a wish
I don't want you to miss.
It's my personal view
And I'll share it with you.

I hope that I will always be,
A woman who is cancer free.
And never do I want to see
Another positive biopsy.

Although no one can predict the future with precision, much is to be said about the factors that seem to influence a positive outcome of the breast cancer experience. Early detection, immediate treatment, coping with aftercare and maintaining a sense of humor all serve to lengthen life and make it more tolerable (if not downright enjoyable) for all involved.

Much is happening in breast cancer research. Discoveries are made every day. Although at this writing, there is no exact method of preventing or curing breast cancer, science has come a long way. Perhaps "the cure" will be discovered tomorrow.

Medical Advances

By Joanna Brell, MD

Even though far from conquered, the advances being made against breast cancer are heartening. More money is being spent on treatments, early detection and prevention than ever before. People are openly discussing the fear and uncertainty associated with breast cancer; husbands, brothers and sons are now showing their concern. There exists more focus on survivorship issues and treating side effects. Quality of life, as well as longevity, are studied. Results will follow when, as a community, we all contribute where we can to improve all aspects of this disease.

So here's to you and all of us who are acquainted with the big Cs. Survive the cancer, tolerate the chemo and move on to the "cure." May you overcome all obstacles to live a long and healthy life.

Appendices

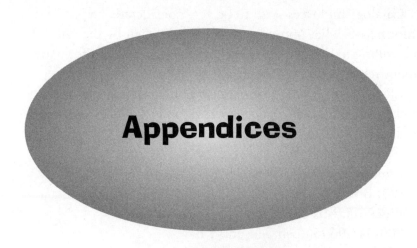

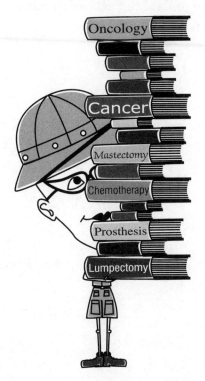

Appendix A: Wig Catalogs

Catalog employees seem to be very considerate, helpful and informative. They appear to sense the stress felt by the caller. They are willing to assist in determining wig size and are informative about returns and exchanges.

I listed Paula Young first because I ordered, returned and exchanged from that catalog. I had good luck with their products and established an instant relationship with their personnel.

Paula Young
P.O. Box 483
Brockton, MA 02303
800-343-9695(open 24 hours / day)
(Offers Christine Jordan, Raquel Welch and Eva Gabor brands, among others, and human hair wigs)

Christine Jordan
P.O. Box 953
S. Easton, MA 02375-9803
800-884-9447 for credit card orders (24 hours / day)
800-490-9447 for customer assistance (during working hours)

Beauty Trends
P.O. Box 9323
Hialeah, FL 33014-9323
800-777-7772
(Offers Cheryl Tiegs wigs for Revlon, Adolfo and Dolly Parton brands among others)

Especially Yours
Dept. B5051
P.O. Box 483
Brockton, MA 02303
888-281-6905, Code B5051X
www.especiallyyours.com/B5051E
(Offers a line of styles from Diahann Carroll)

American Cancer Society "TLC" (Tender Loving Care) Catalog
340 Poplar Street
Hanover, PA 17333-0080
800-850-9445 to order by phone or request a catalog
800-757-9997 to order by fax
http://www.cancer.org to request a catalog on the Internet

All catalog companies feature sales and specials. Some allow returns up to 90 days after purchase. So if the color or size is not right for you, it can be returned and another ordered.

Warming My Head in Style

The jersey turban that I ordered from the American Cancer Society catalog fit snugly on my head so I planned to wear it during the day and evening. But because I was accustomed to some height and fluffiness in my hairstyle, looking like a skinhead flat top bothered me. So I went to my local yardage shop and bought a bag of polyfill, commonly used to fill fabric crafts. I stuffed my jersey turban until it gave me the desired height. After that, I wore my jersey turban more comfortably.

I ordered a terry cloth turban from the American Cancer Society catalog also. Although the terry was soft enough to sleep in, it always ended up on the floor or under one of my pillows midway through the night and I couldn't find it for the other half. So, eventually, I gave up looking. Once it came off, it was off for the night.

The head covering that worked best for me during the night was the green surgical cap I wore to the operating room. Although it was not a number that will be featured in Vogue anytime soon, it was ideal for a head with no hair. It was warm but lightweight and has elastic to hold it in place.

I didn't realize how comfortable this hat would be at the time of the mastectomy because I had not yet experienced hairlessness. But I did think of it at the time of reconstruction. It is always cold in the operating room and I was hairless, so I asked to wear two caps. It was then that I realized how comfortable they were and with two, they even appear a little bouffant. In addition, they stay on during the night better than any other chapeau.

A Deluxe Model

Long after my hair grew in, I received a Miles Kimball catalog advertising a satin sleep cap. It is the same style as the operating room caps but would undoubtedly be more fashionable than the surgical caps. The product number is 464909, the phone number is 702-671-3500, the online number is www.mileskimball.com and the cost is $2.98. Good luck!

Appendix B: Resource Organizations

Clairol Customer Service Hot Line
    800-223-5800
    www.clairol.com

American Cancer Society
    1599 Clifton Road, NE
    Atlanta, GA 30329-4251
Phone: 800-ACS-2345 (800-227-2345)
    www.cancercare.org/bcn/info/brask.html
    www.cancer.org/bottomcancinfo.html

Cancer Care, Inc.
    1180 Avenue of the Americas
    New York, NY 10036-3602
    Phone: 800-813-HOPE (4673)
    Phone: 212-302-2400
    Fax: 212-719-0263
    Email: info@cancercare.org
    www.cancercare.org

National Alliance of Breast Cancer Organizations
    9 E 37th St., 10th Floor
    New York, NY 10016
    Phone: 888-80-NABCO (62226)
    Fax: 212-689-1213
    Email: nabcoinfo@aol.com
    www.nabco.org

National Cancer Institute
    (National Institutes of Health)
    31 Center Drive, MSC 2580
    Bethesda, MD 20892-2580
    www.cancernet.nci.hih.gov

Susan G. Komen Breast Cancer Foundation
5005 LBJ Freeway, Suite 370
Dallas, TX 75244
Phone: 800-IM-AWARE (800-462-9273)
For info on Race for the Cure:
    888-603-RACE (7223)
Fax: 972-855-1605
Email: helpline@komen.org
www.breastcancerinfo.com

Appendix C:
Children's Books

All of these books are stories about a mother who has cancer and may be helpful in teaching children how to talk about and cope with this situation in their own lives.

Kohlenberg, S. (1993). *Sammy's mommy has cancer*. New York: Magination Press

McCue, K., & Bonn, R. (1996). *How to help children through a parent's serious illness* (3rd ed.). NY: St. Martin's Griffin.

Schessel Harpham, W. (1997). *Becky and the worry cup: A children's book about a parent's cancer*. New York: HarperPerennial.

Schessel Harpham, W. (1997). *When a parent has cancer: A guide to caring for your children*. New York: HarperCollins.

Torrey, L. (1998). *Michael's mommy has breast cancer*. Coral Springs, FL: Hibiscus Press.

Winthrop, E. (2000). *Promises*. New York: Clarion Books.

Yaffe, R. S. (1998). *Once upon a hopeful night*. Pittsburgh: Oncology Nursing Press.

Appendix D: Intercultural and Minority Resources

African-American Breast Cancer Alliance
P.O. Box 8981
Minneapolis, MN 55408
Phone: 612-825-3675
Fax: 612-825-3675
(Serves the Twin City area)

Celebrating Life Foundation
P.O. Box 224076
Dallas, TX 75222
Phone: 800-207-0992
Email: clf@cyberramp.net
Web site: www.celebratinglife.org
(For African American women and women of color)

Chinese American Cancer Association
The American Cancer Society, Eastern Division Chinese Unit
41-60 Main Street, #206
Flushing, NY 11355
Phone: 718-886-8890
Fax: 718-886-8981
Web site: www.caca-acs.org/
(For Chinese Americans)

Intercultural Cancer Council
1720 Dryden, Suite C
Houston, TX 77030
Phone: 713-798-5383
Fax: 713-798-3990
Email: icc@bcm.tmc.edu
Web site: icc.bcn.tmc.edu
(Provides information and resources about treatment for minorities)

National Hispanic Leadership on Cancer: En Accion
Baylor College of Medicine, Center for Cancer Control Research
One Baylor Plaza, Suite 924
Houston, TX 77030
Phone: 713-798-4614
Fax: 713-798-3990
Email: celiat@bcm.tmc.edu
Web site: cccr.bcm.tmc.edu/enaccion/
(For Hispanic women and men)

New York Online Access to Health (NOAH)
Web site: www.noah.cuny.edu
(Cancer information in English and Spanish)

Office of Minority Health Resource Center
Rockwall II Building, Suite 1000
5600 Fishers Land
Rockville, MD 20857
Phone: 800-444-6472 / 301-443-5224
Fax: 301-443-8280
Email: 1mosby@omhrc.gov
Web site: www.omhrc.gov
(For information on cancer in minorities)

Appendix E:
Complementary
Treatments for Cancer

There are many supplementary treatments for cancer. The actual effects are not easy to measure. But they can help a person feel better and, taken with traditional cancer treatments, may improve the quality of life. Many of them include healthy principles of living that might enhance all of our lives.

Healing Arts

Art therapy: The use of painting or drawing to express emotion and enhance healing.

Acupuncture: An ancient Chinese practice of piercing certain areas of the body with needles to promote healing and relieve pain.

Garlic: An herb that is thought to trigger the body's defense mechanisms to kill tumor cells.

Herbs and diet supplements: The use of natural substances such as Echinacea and Boost or Ensure to complement food intake and strengthen the body's reserves.

Hypnosis: An induced peaceful state that results in total mind and body relaxation.

Imagery: The process of forming mental pictures of pleasant and soothing scenes to relieve tension.

Macrobiotic diet: A type of vegetarian diet high in grains thought to reestablish balance and harmony in the body.

Massage: The technique of rubbing, kneading and smoothing body muscles to promote relaxation.

Meditation: A technique that achieves the feeling of peace, well-being and renewed energy through relaxation, breathing management and visualization.

Melatonin: A hormone thought to regulate biological rhythms.

Reiki: A Japanese healing tradition that involves hands-on healing touch that is thought to balance the energy that flows through all living things.

Selenium: A mineral that aids the immune system by assisting the body to excrete heavy metals.

Stress management: Includes techniques that are used to control anxiety. Some of these are exercise, deep breathing, spirituality, massage, imagery, yoga, meditation and antianxiety medication.

Stretching and exercising: Certain moves that help tone and relax the body.

T'ai chi: A classical form of Chinese exercise that includes slow, gentle rhythmic movements to produce relaxation and an overall sense of well-being.

Vitamins (particularly A, B complex, C and E): All thought to strengthen the body and promote health. Not all vitamins are water soluble. Check with your doctor before taking more than the recommended daily dose.

Yoga: An ancient system of personal development encompassing body, mind and spirit. It includes meditation, visualization, relaxation, gentle restorative exercises and breathing techniques to induce relaxation.

Programs and Counseling Groups

These programs and groups may be found near your location through the oncology nurse, social service workers at the hospital and community centers and the public relations department of a nearby hospital.

Wellness Programs
> Dressing well after breast surgery
> Makeover techniques to minimize chemo-related appearance changes

Cancer Support Groups
> For men with cancer
> For men whose wives have cancer

For women with breast cancer
For couples: related to breast cancer
For children: when a parent has cancer
For children who have cancer
For parents whose children have cancer
For caregivers of cancer victims

Nutritional Counseling
    Macrobiotic diet
    Melatonin
    Selenium
    Vitamins A, B-Complex, C and E
    Folic acid
    Green tea
    Soy foods
    Antioxidants

Methods of Self-Nurturing
    Get a manicure
    Have a pedicure
    Relax with a good book
    Have tea with a friend
    Indulge in a hot fudge sundae